Diagnostic Issues in Dementia

Advancing the Research Agenda for DSM-V

Diagnostic Issues in Dementia

Advancing the Research Agenda for DSM-V

Edited by

Trey Sunderland, M.D.

Dilip V. Jeste, M.D.

Olusegun Baiyewu, M.D.

Paul J. Sirovatka, M.S.

Darrel A. Regier, M.D., M.P.H.

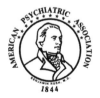

Published by the
American Psychiatric Association
Arlington, Virginia

Copyright © 2007 American Psychiatric Association
ALL RIGHTS RESERVED

Manufactured in the United States of America on acid-free paper
11   10   09   08   07   5   4   3   2   1
First Edition

Typeset in Adobe's Frutiger and AGaramond

American Psychiatric Association
1000 Wilson Boulevard
Arlington, VA 22209-3901
www.psych.org

Library of Congress Cataloging-in-Publication Data
Diagnostic issues in dementia : advancing the research agenda for DSM-V / edited by Trey Sunderland ... [et al.]. — 1st ed.
    p. ; cm.
  Includes bibliographical references and index.
  ISBN 978-0-89042-298-4 (pbk. : alk. paper)
    1. Dementia. 2. Dementia—Research. 3. Mental illness—Treatment.
  I. Sunderland, Trey. II. American Psychiatric Association. [DNLM:
  1. Diagnostic and statistical manual of mental disorders. 5th ed.
  2. Dementia—diagnosis. WM 220 D5355 2007]
  RC521.D5387 2007
  616.8'30072—dc22
                           2007004393

British Library Cataloguing in Publication Data
A CIP record is available from the British Library.

CONTENTS

CONTRIBUTORS

Olusegun Baiyewu, M.D.
Professor of Psychiatry, Department of Psychiatry, College of Medicine, University of Ibadan, Ibadan, Nigeria

Deborah Blacker, M.D., Sc.D.
Director, Gerontology Research Unit, Assistant Vice Chair for Research, Department of Psychiatry, Mass General Hospital/Harvard Medical School; Department of Epidemiology, Harvard School of Public Health, Boston, Massachusetts

John C.S. Breitner, M.D., M.P.H.
Director, Geriatric Research Education and Clinical Center, VA Puget Sound Health Care System; Division of Geriatric Psychiatry, University of Washington School of Medicine, Seattle, Washington

Robert M. Cohen, M.D., Ph.D.
Department of Psychiatry, Cedars-Sinai Medical Center, Los Angeles, California

Harald Hampel, M.D.
Professor of Psychiatry and Director, Alzheimer Memorial Center, Department of Psychiatry, University of Munich, Munich, Germany

Dilip V. Jeste, M.D.
Estelle and Edgar Levi Chair in Aging; Director, Sam and Rose Stein Institute for Research on Aging; Distinguished Professor of Psychiatry and Neurosciences, University of California, San Diego

Daniel S. Kim, M.D.
Geriatric Psychiatry Postdoctoral Fellow, Division of Geriatric Psychiatry, Department of Psychiatry, University of California, San Diego

Simon Lovestone, Ph.D., M.R.C.Psych.
Professor of Old Age Psychiatry, MRC Centre for Neurodegeneration Research, Institute of Psychiatry, Kings College London, London, UK

Thomas W. Meeks, M.D.
Postdoctoral Fellow, Division of Geriatric Psychiatry, Department of Psychiatry, University of California, San Diego

John O'Brien, D.M., M.R.C.Psych.
Wolfson Research Centre, Institute for Ageing and Health, Newcastle General Hospital, Newcastle upon Tyne, UK

Ronald C. Petersen, Ph.D., M.D.
Mayo Clinic College of Medicine, Rochester, Minnesota

Karen T. Putnam, M.S.
Litwin-Zucker Research Center, North Shore–LIJ Health System, Great Neck, New York

Darrel A. Regier, M.D., M.P.H.
Executive Director, American Psychiatric Institute for Research and Education (APIRE), American Psychiatric Association, Arlington, Virginia

Barry Reisberg, M.D.
Professor, Department of Psychiatry and Clinical Director, Silberstein Aging and Dementia Research Center, New York University School of Medicine, New York, New York

Mary Sano, Ph.D.
Alzheimer Disease Research Center of Mount Sinai School of Medicine, New York, New York; James J. Peters VAMC, Bronx, New York

Norman Sartorius, M.D., Ph.D.
Adjunct Professor of Psychiatry, Washington University, St. Louis, Missouri; Visiting Professor, University of London, Prague, Beijing, and Zagreb

Paul J. Sirovatka, M.S.
Associate Director for Research Policy Analysis, Division of Research/American Psychiatric Institute for Research and Education (APIRE), Arlington, Virginia

Gary W. Small, M.D.
Parlow-Solomon Professor on Aging; Professor of Psychiatry & Biobehavioral Sciences; Director, UCLA Center on Aging; Director, Memory & Aging Research Center, University of California, Los Angeles, California

Trey Sunderland, M.D.
National Institute of Mental Health, Bethesda, Maryland

Masatoshi Takeda, M.D., Ph.D.
Chairman and Professor, Department of Clinical Neuroscience, Osaka University Graduate School of Medicine, Osaka, Japan

Robert D. Terry, M.D.
Professor Emeritus, Department of Neurosciences, University of California, San Diego, California

George S. Zubenko, M.D., Ph.D.
Professor, Department of Psychiatry, University of Pittsburgh, Pittsburgh, Pennsylvania

DISCLOSURE STATEMENT

The research conference series that produced this monograph is supported with funding from the U.S. National Institutes of Health (NIH) Grant No. U13-MH067855 (Principal Investigator: Darrel A. Regier, M.D., M.P.H.). The National Institute of Mental Health (NIMH), the National Institute on Drug Abuse (NIDA), and the National Institute on Alcohol Abuse and Alcoholism (NIAAA) jointly support this cooperative research planning conference project. The Workgroup/Conference on Diagnostic Issues in Dementia is not part of the official revision process for the *Diagnostic and Statistical Manual of Mental Disorders,* Fifth Edition (DSM-V), but rather is a separate, rigorous research planning initiative meant to inform revisions of psychiatric diagnostic classification systems. No private-industry sources provide funding for the research review.

Coordination and oversight of the overall research review, publicly titled "The Future of Psychiatric Diagnosis: Refining the Research Agenda," is provided by an Executive Steering Committee composed of representatives of the several entities that are cooperatively sponsoring the NIH-funded project. Present and former members are as follows:

- *American Psychiatric Institute for Research and Education*—Darrel A. Regier, M.D., M.P.H.; support staff: William E. Narrow, M.D., M.P.H., Maritza Rubio-Stipec, Sci.D., Paul Sirovatka, M.S., Jennifer Shupinka, Rocio Salvador, and Kristin Edwards
- *World Health Organization*—Benedetto Saraceno, M.D., and Norman Sartorius, M.D., Ph.D. (consultant)
- *National Institutes of Health*—Michael Kozak, Ph.D. (NIMH), Wilson Compton, M.D. (NIDA), and Bridget Grant, Ph.D. (NIAAA); NIMH grant project officers have included Bruce Cuthbert, Ph.D., Lisa Colpe, Ph.D., Michael Kozak, Ph.D., and Karen H. Bourdon, M.A.
- *Columbia University*—Michael B. First, M.D. (consultant)

The following contributors to this book have indicated financial interests in or other affiliations with a commercial supporter, a manufacturer of a commercial product, a provider of a commercial service, a nongovernmental organization, and/or a government agency, as listed below:

Robert M. Cohen, M.D., Ph.D.—Research unit that author directs currently uses funds from projects sponsored by Alkermes, Johnson & Johnson, Solvay Pharmaceuticals, AstraZeneca, Janssen, Organon, NARSAD, Sepracor, Forest Research Institute, Cyberonics, Aspect Medical Systems, National Center for Complementary and Alternative Medicine (NCCAM), and the National Institute of Mental Health (NIMH). In addition to the operational funds for conducting research described above, the author receives salary support for performing trials from Forest Research Institute, Cyberonics, Aspect Medical Systems, NCCAM, and NIMH.

Dilip V. Jeste, M.D.—The author's work in this volume was supported, in part, by National Institute of Mental Health Grant MH66248 and by the Department of Veteran Affairs. *Consultant:* Otsuka, Bristol-Myers Squibb, Janssen, Solvay, and Wyeth Pharmaceuticals. AstraZeneca, Bristol-Myers Squibb, Eli Lilly, and Janssen supply free medications for the author's NIMH-funded R01: "Metabolic Effects of Newer Antipsychotics in Older Patients."

Simon Lovestone, Ph.D., M.R.C.Psych.—Collaborations with GlaxoSmithKline, Proteome Sciences, Celera. *Consultant:* Neuropharma, Neurochem, MSD, Eisai. *Funds for speaking/lectures:* Lundbeck. Intellectual property interests in biomarkers for AD managed by King's College London Enterprises.

John O'Brien, D.M., M.R.C.Psych.—*Consultant:* GE Healthcare. The author has accepted lecture fees for speaking from Pfizer/Eisai, Shire, Lundbeck and Novartis. The author has attended advisory boards for Novartis, Lundbeck, Pfizer/Eisai, Shire, and GE Healthcare.

Ronald C. Petersen, Ph.D., M.D.—*Consultant:* Elan Pharmaceuticals (Chair of Safety Monitoring Committee); GE Healthcare. *Lecturer:* Servier.

Darrel A. Regier, M.D., M.P.H.—The author, as Executive Director of American Psychiatric Institute for Research and Education (APIRE), oversees all federal and industry -sponsored research and research training grants in APIRE but receives no external salary funding or honoraria from any government or industry sources.

Barry Reisberg, M.D.—The author receives research grant support from U.S. governmental, foundation, private, and industrial sources. These include the National Institute on Aging (NIA) and the General Clinical Research Center Program of the U.S. National Institutes of Health (NIH), U.S. DHHS Administration on Aging (AOA), the Fisher Center for Alzheimer's Disease Research Foundation, grants from Mr. Leonard Litwin, the Hagedorn Foundation, the Harry and Jennie Slayton Foundation, the Sonya Samberg Family Trust, the Forest Research Institute, and Myriad Pharmaceuticals. He is a consultant on a grant from the National Institute of Child Health and Human Development of the NIH and a grant from the government of Upper Austria. He directs a Clinical Research Fellowship supported in part by Forest Laboratories. He is a consultant for Johnson & Johnson. He has received symposium support, travel support, speaker fees and/or honoraria, or consultant fees in the past few years (2005 to present) from Janssen Pharmaceutica, Forest Laboratories, Merz GmbH, Eurand, Glaxo-Smith Kline, Lundbeck Pharmaceuticals, the Lundbeck Institute, the State University of New York at Stony Brook School of Medicine, Saint Vincent Catholic Medical Centers (New York), the University of Alsasua (Navarra, Spain) , the American Conference on Psychiatric Disorders, the Morbus Alzheimer Society (Bad Ischl, Austria), the Southeast Missouri Hospital Foundation (Missouri), in coordination with Southeast Missouri State University and the Alzheimer's Association, Cape Girardeau (Missouri), the Maria Wolff Foundation (Madrid, Spain), American Psychiatric Institute for Research and Education, the International Psychogeriatric Association, and the Turkish Psychiatric Association. He has played a role in the development and/or naming of some of the concepts discussed in the chapter (e.g., mild cognitive impairment; see relevant citations in the chapter), and he is the developer and copyright holder of some of the assessment instruments discussed in this chapter, as cited in the chapter references. Dr. Reisberg, in association with co-inventors, holds U.S. patents for: "method for the assessment of severe dementia," "system for diagnosis and staging of dementia by neurologic examination," "staging of dementia severity by joint function examination," "method for diagnosis of incontinence of corticocerebral origin by neurologic examination," "method and apparatus employing motor measures for early diagnosis and staging of dementia," and "management, care, and treatment of Alzheimer's disease and related dementias."

Norman Sartorius, M.D., Ph.D.—The author has served as a consultant to Eli Lilly, Janssen, Lundbeck, Servier, and Wyeth and received a fee for participating in symposia organized by Eli Lilly, Janssen, and Pfizer. He has not received any funds for research or staff or fees for organizing education. The author does not own shares of any organization that may give rise to a conflict of interest.

Gary W. Small, M.D.—The University of California, Los Angeles, owns a U.S. patent (6,274,119) entitled "Methods for Labeling β-Amyloid Plaques and Neurofibrillary Tangles," which has been licensed to Siemens. Dr. Small is among the inventors, has received royalties, and will receive royalties on future sales. Dr. Small reports having served as a consultant and/or having received lecture fees from Abbott, Brainstorming Co., Dakim, Eisai, Forest Laboratories, Myriad Genetics, Novartis, Ortho-McNeil, Pfizer, Radica, Servier, and Siemens. Dr. Small also reports having received stock options from Dakim and having received a grant from GlaxoSmithKline.

Trey Sunderland, M.D.—The author reports no support that presents a conflict of interest in the past 2 years. Previous support includes consulting and honorarium from Lundbeck, Abbott, Bristol-Myers Squibb, Pfizer, and Janssen.

George S. Zubenko, M.D., Ph.D.—University of Pittsburgh (salaried faculty member). National Institute of Mental Health/National Institutes of Health (grants and reviewer, including MH069629 to Partners Healthcare/Harvard Medical School). Mutual funds.

The following contributors to this book do not have any conflicts of interest to disclose:

Olusegun Baiyewu, M.D.
Deborah Blacker, M.D., Sc.D.
John C.S. Breitner, M.D., M.P.H.
Harald Hampel, M.D.
Daniel S. Kim, M.D.
Thomas W. Meeks, M.D.
Mary Sano, Ph.D.
Paul J. Sirovatka, M.S.
Masatoshi Takeda, M.D., Ph.D.
Robert D. Terry, M.D.

FOREWORD

Darrel A. Regier, M.D., M.P.H.

Diagnostic Issues in Dementia: Advancing the Research Agenda for DSM-V continues a series of volumes that collectively summarize an international research-planning project undertaken to assess the status of scientific knowledge that is relevant to psychiatric classification systems and to generate specific recommendations for research to advance that knowledge base. The conference series, titled "The Future of Psychiatric Diagnosis: Refining the Research Agenda," is being convened by the American Psychiatric Association (APA) with the collaboration of the World Health Organization (WHO) and the U.S. National Institutes of Health (NIH), with NIH funding.

The APA/WHO/NIH conference series and monographs represent key elements in an extensive research review process designed to set the stage for the fifth edition of the *Diagnostic and Statistical Manual of Mental Disorders* (DSM-V). In its entirety, the project entails 11 work groups focused on a specific diagnostic topic or category. The monographs—and, in most instances, prior publication of the work-group/conference proceedings in the peer-reviewed literature—reflect the APA's efforts to ensure that information and recommendations developed as part of this process are available to scientific groups who are concurrently updating other national and international classifications of mental and behavioral disorders.

Within the APA, the American Psychiatric Institute for Research and Education (APIRE), under the direction of Darrel A. Regier, M.D., M.P.H., holds lead responsibility for organizing and administering the diagnosis research planning conferences. Co-sponsors, and members of the Executive Steering Committee for the series, include representatives of the WHO's Department of Mental Health and Substance Abuse and of three NIH institutes that are jointly funding the project: National Institute of Mental Health (NIMH), National Institute on Drug Abuse (NIDA), and National Institute on Alcohol Abuse and Alcoholism (NIAAA).

APA published the fourth edition of DSM in 1994, and a text revision appeared in 2000. Planning for the fifth edition, however, began in 1999 with a collaboration between APA and the NIMH designed to stimulate research that would address identified opportunities in psychiatric nosology. A first product of this joint venture was preparation of six white papers that proposed broad-brush recommendations for research in key areas; topics included developmental issues, gaps in the current classification, disability and impairment, neuroscience, nomenclature, and cross-cultural issues. Each team that developed a paper included at least one liaison member from NIMH, with the intent—largely realized—that these members would integrate many of the work groups' recommendations into NIMH research support programs. These white papers were published in *A Research Agenda for DSM-V* (Kupfer et al. 2002). This volume has been followed more recently by a second compilation of white papers, edited by Narrow and colleagues,[1] that outline diagnosis-related research needs in the areas of gender, infants and children, and geriatric populations.

As a second phase of planning, the APA leadership envisioned a series of international research planning conferences that would address specific diagnostic topics in greater depth, with conference proceedings serving as resource documents for groups involved in the official DSM-V revision process. A prototype symposium on mood disorders was held in conjunction with the XII World Congress of Psychiatry in Yokohama, Japan, in late 2002. Presentations addressed diverse topics in depression-related research, including preclinical animal models, genetics, pathophysiology, functional imaging, clinical treatment, epidemiology, prevention, medical comorbidity, and public health implications of the full spectrum of mood disorders. This pilot meeting underscored the importance of structuring multidisciplinary research planning conferences in a manner that would force interaction among investigators from different fields and elicit a sharp focus on the diagnostic implications of recent and planned research. Lessons learned in Yokohama guided development of the proposal for the cooperative research planning conference grant that NIMH awarded to APIRE in 2003, with substantial additional funding support from NIDA and NIAAA. The conferences funded under the grant are the basis for this monograph series and represent a second major phase in the scientific review and planning for DSM-V.

Finally, a third major component of advance planning has been the DSM-V Prelude Project, an APA-sponsored Web site designed to keep the DSM user community and the public informed about research and other activities related to the fifth edition of the manual. An "outreach" section of the site permits interested parties to submit comments about problems with DSM-IV and suggestions for DSM-V. All suggestions are being entered into the DSM-V Prelude database for eventual referral to the appropriate DSM-V Work Groups. This site and associated links can be accessed at www.dsm5.org.

The conferences that constitute the core activity of the second phase of preparation have multiple aims. One is to promote international collaboration among members of the scientific community in order to increase the likelihood of developing a future DSM that is unified with other international classifications. A second is to stimulate the empirical research necessary to allow informed decision making regarding diagnostic deficiencies identified in DSM-IV. A third is to facilitate the development of broadly agreed upon criteria that researchers worldwide can use in planning and conducting future research into the etiology and pathophysiology of mental disorders. Challenging as it is, this last objective reflects widespread agreement in the field that the well-established reliability and clinical utility of prior DSM classifications must be matched in the future by a renewed focus on the validity of diagnoses.

Given the vision of an ultimately unified international classification system, members of the Executive Steering Committee have attached high priority to assuring the participation of investigators from all parts of the world in the project. Toward this end, each conference in the series will have two co-chairs, drawn respectively from the United States and a country other than the United States; approximately half of the 25 experts invited to each working conference are from outside the United States; and half of the conferences are being convened outside the United States.

Three leaders in the field of dementia research—Trey Sunderland, M.D., of the National Institutes of Health; Dilip V. Jeste, M.D., of the University of California, San Diego; and Olusegun Baiyewu, M.D., of the University of Ibadan, Nigeria—agreed to organize and co-chair the Dementia Work Group and conference, which convened in Geneva, Switzerland, in September 2005. The co-chairs worked closely with the APA/WHO/NIH Executive Steering Committee to identify and enlist a stellar roster of participants for the conference.

Papers from the conference on dementia initially appeared in the *Journal of Geriatric Psychiatry and Neurology* (Vol. 19, No. 3, September 2006). In addition, a summary report of the conference is available online at www.dsm5.org.

The American Psychiatric Association greatly appreciates the contributions of all participants in the dementia research planning work group and the interest of our broader audience in this topic.

Reference

1.   Narrow WN, First MB, Sirovatka P, Regier DA (eds): Age and Gender Considerations in Psychiatric Diagnosis: A Research Agenda for DSM-V. Arlington, VA, American Psychiatric Association, 2007

PREFACE[1]

Modern Diagnostic Approaches in Dementia: On the Cusp of Change

Trey Sunderland, M.D.

Change in personal habits is difficult enough for most people, because well-worn patterns beckon with comfortable familiarity. Change in professional habits, such as those represented in our basic diagnostic nomenclature, is perhaps even more vexing to accomplish smoothly, because consensus is attempted among numerous people across complex and often controversial topics. The chapters in this volume, first published in an issue of the *Journal of Geriatric Psychiatry and Neurology* (Vol. 19, No. 3, September 2006), are focused on some of the upcoming changes anticipated for the dementias as the American Psychiatric Association prepares for publication of the *Diagnostic and Statistical Manual of Mental Disorders,* 5th Edition (DSM-V). Prompted by the American Psychiatric Institute for Research and Education and supported by a multi-institutional grant from the National Institute of Mental Health, National Institute on Drug Abuse, and National Institute on Alcohol Abuse and Alcoholism, a series of meetings have been planned over the next several years to begin that process of diagnostic change for the many psychiatric illnesses. The chapters in this book reflect that nascent effort toward a new diagnostic nomenclature in the dementia field.

Not all important diagnostic issues in dementia can possibly be covered in a relatively brief compendium, but this collection represents a considered effort. Robert Terry (see Chapter 1) starts the process with the all-important neuropathological criteria of Alzheimer's disease (AD) and the aging brain, citing the expanding database for the non-AD dementias. John Breitner (see Chapter 2) next provides an insightful assessment of the extant epidemiological literature and points out the challenges in-

---

[1]This preface is reprinted from Sunderland T: "Modern Diagnostic Approaches in Dementia: On the Cusp of Change." *Journal of Geriatric Psychiatry and Neurology* 19:123–124, 2006. Used with permission.

volved with even minor changes in our general definition of dementia. Barry Reisberg and Norman Sartorius (see Chapter 3) follow with a scholarly review of the diagnostic nomenclature across the existing criteria, with numerous critiques and suggestions for future research. Ronald Petersen and John O'Brien (see Chapter 4) outline the growing evidence for mild cognitive impairment (MCI) as an identifiable entity and make a strong case for the possible inclusion of amnestic MCI in the next iteration of DSM. Mary Sano (see Chapter 5) then highlights the current neuropsychological profiling that serves as the centerpiece of the diagnostic criteria for dementia and suggests that new instruments evaluating even broader aspects of cognition, including executive function, will be important in helping identify dementia at an earlier stage of development. Dilip Jeste and colleagues (see Chapter 6) give us a thorough review of the various neuropsychiatric syndromes associated with dementia, emphasizing the need for greater diagnostic clarity to help focus appropriate therapy in this area of increased burden for patients and family caregivers. Trey Sunderland and colleagues (see Chapter 7) next describe the burgeoning literature on biomarkers in AD and suggest that certain of these biomarkers, particularly the cerebrospinal fluid measures of β-amyloid and tau, may already be appropriate for inclusion in our diagnostic criteria. Gary Small (see Chapter 8) emphasizes the current diagnostic utility of specific imaging modalities, including fluorodeoxyglucose positron emission tomography scans, and suggests that combining imaging methods with expanding ligand technology or markers of genetic predisposition might further enhance diagnostic accuracy. Finally, in a sobering reminder of the limits of the current genetic knowledge base and the great heterogeneity of the dementias, Deborah Blacker and Simon Lovestone (see Chapter 9) review the tremendous explosion of information in this field and conclude that with the exception of the rare Mendelian disorders, genetic profiles are not yet ready to make substantial contributions to nosology.

Each chapter describes a piece of the dementia diagnostic story, but these authors' views cannot be considered in isolation. There is a vast and expanding literature related to the dementias, especially with respect to AD, and the field is still evolving rapidly. Given the associated but still generally nonspecific biological mechanisms underlying these syndromes, new scientific developments in any one of a thousand research centers around the world might immediately affect the interpretations and considerations of our expert authors. With that proviso in mind, we must be cautious in making any overly dogmatic proclamations about firm diagnostic criteria at this time. Even though the dementia field has some of the most definitive clinicopathological findings, clear clinical patterns of cognitive and behavioral abnormalities, absolute genetic mutations for a fraction of the disorders and at least one prominent genetic association marker, and emerging neuroimaging and other biomarkers, we are dealing mostly with clinical syndromes and still use clinical diagnostic criteria established at consensus conferences. It is with that spirit of scientific humility that we present these contributions with research suggestions for consideration in the upcoming DSM-V process.

1

ALZHEIMER'S DISEASE AND THE AGING BRAIN

Robert D. Terry, M.D.

Until a few years ago, we knew of only two neurodegenerative forms of dementia: Alzheimer's and Pick's. They were often spoken of in the same breath, as if they were of equal frequency. We now know that Pick's disease, as diagnosed by histologic criteria, is only about 1/50th as frequent as Alzheimer's disease (AD). However, in the past couple of decades, further dementias have been recognized and have added to the complexity. Among these are Lewy body dementia, which most commonly occurs with AD but sometimes occurs alone, and frontotemporal disorder, which is a group subsuming Pick's disease and the dementia associated with Parkinson's disease and with amyotrophic lateral sclerosis. Those rare disorders associated with prions are not to be considered here. The skills required for accurate clinical differentiation among all these dementias are best acquired by association with a large autopsy experience.

The following nosology is based on pathology:

- Alzheimer's disease: 60%
- Lewy body variant (of AD): 20%
- Pure Lewy body: 5%

This chapter is reprinted from Terry RD: "Alzheimer's Disease and the Aging Brain." *Journal of Geriatric Psychiatry and Neurology* 19:125–128, 2006. Used with permission.

- Frontotemporal (including Pick's): 5%
- Vascular: 5%
- Miscellaneous: 5%

Thus, AD is primarily involved in about 80% of dementia cases. About 2% of patients with AD are the unfortunate carriers of one of the three causal dominant AD genes on chromosome 21,[1] chromosome 14,[2] or chromosome 1.[3] Almost all the other 98% are sporadic; that is, they do not carry a dominant gene for the disease but may well have an allele such as *APOE* ε4 that increases the risk of getting AD.[4] The frequency of AD increases as a function of age, so one might well consider the cerebral changes that occur with normal aging also as risk factors.

Normal Aging

A few plaques may well be present in the neocortex and hippocampal-entorhinal region of any cognitively normal elderly person. Neurofibrillary tangles (NFTs) are extremely rare in the neocortex of normal persons, but again a few may be present in the medial temporal area. Plaques and tangles, the classic lesions of AD, are described in detail later in this chapter.

Cortical neurons have been counted by three methods beginning in the early years of the twentieth century. Before about 1955, these efforts involved simply counting the cells as identified with the light microscope. One well-known report stated that the neocortex loses significant numbers, especially among the small neurons.[5] Computerized image analysis became available in the 1970s, and this relatively expensive apparatus permitted measurement of cell size as well as cell number. The surprising results demonstrated that the larger neurons shrink into the smaller class, but without a total loss.[6] The current standard requires the use of stereology, by which a sample of cells is selected by their coincidence with a superimposed pattern.[7] The results are essentially identical to those accomplished by image analysis; that is, the density of neurons (cells per unit area or volume of tissue) is not diminished in the course of normal aging. Overall, it should be kept in mind that the cortex does shrink a little, so that the total number of neocortical nerve cells must slightly decline correspondingly.

Enumeration of synapses has been accomplished by reacting the tissue sections with antisynaptophysin, which reacts with the indicated protein in the membrane of synaptic vesicles in the terminal axonal bouton.[8] With appropriate illumination, each presynaptic bouton is identified by the presence of a luminescent dot (a cluster of synaptic vesicles) that can be quantified with computerized confocal microscopy.[9] This technique indicates a significant loss of synapses in normal aging despite the well-maintained neuronal number.[10] The diminished number of synapses may be the cause or the result of neuronal shrinkage and may also be responsible for those cognitive changes found in normally aging elderly persons. Unfortunately, there has not been any attempt to correlate cognitive ability with synapse concentration in normal aging.

These findings probably explain why patients with early-onset AD display higher concentrations of lesions than do older patients. The presentation of any disease depends on the disease process and also on the premorbid condition of the affected organ. The young patient prior to onset of the disease has a full complement of synapses and thus must lose more before becoming symptomatic. The older patient, having lost synapses by the time of onset, will display symptoms with relatively less further decrement caused by the disease.

Structural Changes in Alzheimer's Disease

NFTs, first described by Alzheimer himself,[11] are significantly present in the entorhinal cortex and hippocampus as well as in the neocortex in varying but usually prominent concentrations. For example, the primary visual cortex (Brodmann area 17) has a lesser concentration than the adjacent associated area 18, which in turn projects to more distant cortical areas that have still greater numbers of NFTs.[12] The primary motor cortex is also less affected by tangles. These lesions lie inside the cytoplasm of larger neurons and are stained with Congo red and certain other amyloid stains, which gave rise to the confusion of their chemical nature with that of amyloid. However, Margolis[13] demonstrated that the tangle was not amyloid in 1959. Electron microscopy published by Kidd[14] in 1963 showed that the NFT is made up of paired helical filaments (PHFs), with each member filament being 100 Å thick with a half twist every 800 Å. In 1985, the Belgian neurologist Brion and colleagues[15] proved that the PHFs are made up of tau protein, which is a normal neuronal constituent. More recently, it was shown that the tau in the tangles is abnormally hyperphosphorylated.[16]

Neocortical tangles are very rare in normal cognition. Braak and Braak[17] established a classification of the clinicopathological severity of the disease based on the spread of tangles from the mesial temporal region throughout the cortex.

One problem with this concept is that beyond the age of 70 years and increasingly in greater age, we find entirely typical AD without cortical tangles. Alzheimer's second case, published in 1910 and recently reexamined,[18] was of this type. We had previously found the phenomenon in about 20% of our autopsied cases involving individuals over 70 years of age at time of death.[19] One might wonder whether there is an agent in elderly people that blocks the pairing of hyperphosphorylated filaments or whether there is less phosphorylation. In any case, these patients are just as demented as their coevals with neocortical tangles.

The mass of PHFs nearly fills the cytoplasm of affected neurons, which in the neocortex are mostly glutamatergic. Extracellular tangles are frequently found in the medial temporal region but are quite rare in the neocortex. In either case, these pathological markers reflect neuronal death, which also occurs frequently in the absence of PHFs.

Senile or neuritic plaques are ubiquitous throughout the neocortex as well as in the mesial temporal region. Plaques had been reported[20] well before Alzheimer, but their significance was not recognized. The lesions measure up to about 150 μm and are roughly spherical. Light microscopy with amyloid stains such as Congo red or thioflavin reveals a core of extracellular, fibrillar amorphous material. Divry[21] was the first to recognize that the amorphous material in the plaques is indeed amyloid. The amyloid is surrounded by silver-stained neurites in a sort of halo. Fibrous astrocytes can be discerned on the periphery. Electron microscopy[22] confirmed the presence of amyloid in the form of 95-Å filaments. The neurites in the plaque were seen to be bulbous, dystrophic unmyelinated axons and dendrites containing dense bodies (lysosomes),[23] filaments, and PHFs. Synaptic terminals are sometimes present.[24] Activated microglia are prominent in the plaque in intimate relation to the amyloid and also are scattered throughout the neuropil, perhaps in response to degenerating synapses.

The walls of small arteries and arterioles are often infiltrated by amyloid, which is usually located in the vascular media among the smooth muscle cells. The change is very rarely occlusive, but these vessels do occasionally give rise to hemorrhage. The affected vessels are usually confined to the leptomeninges and cortex but are very occasionally in the subcortical white matter of the centrum ovale. When these latter vessels bleed, the hemorrhage is often in superficial locations that are relatively rare compared with the usual hypertensive hemorrhagic stroke not associated with amyloid.

Neurons are extensively lost from neocortex, hippocampus, and the entorhinal region.[25] The basal nucleus of Meynert lying ventral to the pallidum is severely affected by cell loss as well as by plaques and tangles.[26] Normally, these neurons are the major source of acetylcholine, which would be widely distributed to hippocampus and cortex but which is characteristically deficient in the disease.[27] Image analysis counts in midfrontal area 46 (Brodmann), superior temporal area 38/22, and inferior parietal area 39 in elderly patients with dementia demonstrated a decrease of about 30% compared with age-matched normally functioning elders.[25] The loss is nearly twice as severe in younger, presenile patients.

The loss of neocortical synapses in AD is about 45%,[28] which is significantly greater than the loss of the cell bodies (about 30%),[25] but, as in normal aging, we do not know whether dendritic spines decrease concurrently with or even before the axonal decrement. Golgi studies of some years ago clearly showed the dendritic atrophy and loss of spines, but these changes could not be quantified, nor were they correlated with loss of presynaptic boutons.[29] An article by a prominent investigator usually involved in the study of amyloid is titled "Alzheimer's Disease Is a Synaptic Failure."[30]

There has been a recent revival (see the article by Alvarez[31]) of interest in ischemia as a causal phenomenon in AD. Infarcts are, however, not at all commonly found in the Alzheimer's brain, and the arteries are actually usually remarkably free of atheromatous change. The coincidence of functional abnormalities of the heart simultaneous with increasing dementia cannot be ignored, but the connection is not apparent to this observer.

Correlations and Conclusions

In 1968, Blessed, Tomlinson, and Roth[32] published their quantitative studies of neocortical plaques and correlated those counts with Blessed's test of cognition. They reported a strong correlation, which may well have given rise to the widespread concept that amyloid causes dementia and is at the root of Alzheimer's disease.[33] The trouble with that statistical plot[32] is that many cases fell on or near the vertical axis (dementia without plaques), whereas many other cases were on or near the horizontal axis (plaques without dementia). In neither of these groups was AD really present, and the remaining cases displayed a weak or nonsignificant correlation. Our own attempts to duplicate the Newcastle study with only proven cases of AD never came close to showing strong relationships. Most investigators today accept that soluble, oligomeric Aβ peptide from the amyloid precursor protein on chromosome 21 is the principal toxic agent rather than the fibrillar extracellular amyloid, which appears to be relatively inert. Quite recently, Aβ oligomers have been found in presynaptic boutons and in terminal axons.[34] The neuron counts provide moderately strong correlates with cognition, but strongest of all the structural correlations with severity of cognitive loss is that of presynaptic boutons as measured with the antisynaptophysin reaction quantified by confocal microscopy.[28] The synaptic loss causes disconnections between parts of the brain and between individual neurons or groups of neurons, thus providing an entirely rational explanation of dementia.

By way of hopes for the future, I would like to see far more autopsies done on patients whose diagnosis of one or another organic dementia is made by psychiatrists. We at the University of California, San Diego, have an autopsy rate of 80%–85% on dementia cases, so it can be done if the physicians and staff are interested in improving their diagnostic skills as well as providing material for research. Special histologic methods will be required to recognize certain types of dementia on autopsy specimens. On a different level, there should be developed a method for the in vivo determination of synaptic population density. This would provide a strong correlate with cognition in normal aging and dementia. The technique might be analogous to the Pittsburgh method for recognizing the amyloid of plaques with positron emission tomography.[35] It is to be noted that this plaque amyloid is not the cause of neuronal or synaptic loss, as is the oligomeric Aβ, which is not recognized by this method. Nevertheless, the technique is useful in that in most cases there is a fair correlation between plaque intensity and disease state.

References

1. Tanzi RE, Gusella JF, Watkins PC, et al: Amyloid beta protein gene: cDNA, mRNA distribution, and genetic linkage near the Alzheimer locus. Science 235:880–884, 1987.

2. St George-Hyslop P, Haines J, Rogaev E, et al: Genetic evidence for a novel familial Alzheimer's disease locus on chromosome 14. Nat Genet 2:330–334, 1992.

3. Price DL, Tanzi RE, Borchelt DR, et al: Alzheimer's disease: genetic studies and transgenic models. Annu Rev Genet 32:461–493, 1998.

4. Strittmatter WJ, Saunders AM, Schmechel D, et al: Apolipoprotein E: high-avidity binding to beta-amyloid and increased frequency of type 4 allele in late-onset familial Alzheimer disease. Proc Natl Acad Sci U S A 90:1977–1981, 1993.

5. Brody H: Organization of the cerebral cortex, III: a study of aging in the human cerebral cortex. J Comp Neurol 102:511–516, 1955.

6. Terry RD, DeTeresa R, Hansen LA: Neocortical cell counts in normal human adult aging. Ann Neurol 21:530–539, 1987.

7. Gomez-Isla T, Hollister R, West H, et al: Neuronal loss correlates with but exceeds neurofibrillary tangles in Alzheimer's disease. Ann Neurol 41:17–24, 1997.

8. Jahn R, Schiebler W, Ouimet C, et al: A 38,000-dalton membrane protein (p38) present in synaptic vesicles. Proc Natl Acad Sci U S A 82:4137–4141, 1985.

9. Masliah E, Terry RD, Alford M, et al: Cortical and subcortical patterns of synaptophysinlike immunoreactivity in Alzheimer's disease. Am J Pathol 138:235–246, 1991.

10. Masliah E, Mallory M, Hansen L, et al: Quantitative synaptic alterations in the human neocortex during normal aging. Neurology 43:192–197, 1993.

11. Alzheimer A: Über eine eigenartige Erkrankung der Hirnrinde. Allgemeine Zeitschrift für Psychiatrie und psychisch-gerichtliche Medizin 64:146–148, 1907.

12. Lewis DA, Campbell MJ, Terry RD, et al: Laminar and regional distributions of neurofibrillary tangles and neuritic plaques in Alzheimer's disease: a quantitative study of visual and auditory cortices. J Neurosci 7:1799–1808, 1987.

13. Margolis G: Senile cerebral disease: a critical survey of traditional concepts based upon observations with newer techniques. Lab Invest 8:335–370, 1959.

14. Kidd M: Paired helical filaments in electron microscopy of Alzheimer's disease. Nature 197:192–193, 1963.

15. Brion JP, Passareiro H, Nunez J, et al: Mise en évidence immunologique de la protéine tau au niveau des lésions de dégénérescence neurofibrillaire de la maladie d'Alzheimer. Arch Biol (Brux) 95:229–235, 1985.

16. Grundke-Iqbal I, Iqbal K, Tung YC, et al: Abnormal phosphorylation of the microtubule-associated protein tau (tau) in Alzheimer cytoskeletal pathology. Proc Natl Acad Sci U S A 83:4913–4917, 1986.

17. Braak H, Braak E: Neuropathological staging of Alzheimer-related changes. Acta Neuropathol (Berl) 82:239–259, 1991.

18. Graeber MB, Kosel S, Egensperger R, et al: Rediscovery of the case described by Alois Alzheimer in 1911: historical, histological and molecular genetic analysis. Neurogenetics 1:73–80, 1997.

19. Terry RD, Hansen LA, DeTeresa R, et al: Senile dementia of the Alzheimer type without neocortical neurofibrillary tangles. J Neuropathol Exp Neurol 46:262–268, 1987.

20. Blocq P, Marinesco G: Sur les lésions et la pathogénie de l'épilepsie dite essentielle. La Semaine médicale 12:445–446, 1892.
21. Divry P: Etude histochimique des plaques séniles. Journal belge de neurologie et de psychiatrie 27:643–657, 1927.
22. Terry RD, Gonatas NK, Weiss M: Ultrastructural studies in Alzheimer's presenile dementia. Am J Pathol 44:269–297, 1964.
23. Suzuki K, Terry RD: Fine structural localization of acid phosphatase in senile plaques in Alzheimer's presenile dementia. Acta Neuropathol (Berl) 8:276–284, 1967.
24. Gonatas NK, Anderson W, Evangelista I: The contribution of altered synapses in the senile plaque: an electron microscopic study in Alzheimer's dementia. J Neuropathol Exp Neurol 26:25–39, 1967.
25. Terry RD, Peck A, DeTeresa R, et al: Some morphometric aspects of the brain in senile dementia of the Alzheimer type. Ann Neurol 10:184–192, 1981.
26. Whitehouse PJ, Price DL, Struble RG, et al: Alzheimer's disease and senile dementia: loss of neurons in the basal forebrain. Science 215:1237–1239, 1982.
27. Davies P, Maloney AJ: Selective loss of central cholinergic neurons in Alzheimer's disease (letter). Lancet 2:1403, 1976.
28. Terry RD, Masliah E, Salmon DP, et al: Physical basis of cognitive alterations in Alzheimer's disease: synapse loss is the major correlate of cognitive impairment. Ann Neurol 30:572–580, 1991.
29. Scheibel AB: Structural aspects of the aging brain: spine systems and the dendritic arbor, in Alzheimer's Disease Dementia and Related Disorders. Edited by Katzman R, Terny RD, Bick PL. New York, Raven, 1978, pp 353–373.
30. Selkoe DJ: Alzheimer's disease is a synaptic failure. Science 298:789–791, 2002.
31. Alvarez WC: Cerebral arteriosclerosis with small, commonly unrecognized apoplexies. Geriatrics 1:189–216, 1946.
32. Blessed G, Tomlinson BE, Roth M: The association between quantitative measures of dementia and of senile change in the cerebral grey matter of elderly subjects. Br J Psychiatry 114:797–811, 1968.
33. Hardy JA, Higgins GA: Alzheimer's disease: the amyloid cascade hypothesis. Science 256:184–185, 1992.
34. Kokubo H, Kayed R, Glabe CG, et al: Soluble Abeta oligomers ultrastructurally localize to cell processes and might be related to synaptic dysfunction in Alzheimer's disease brain. Brain Res 1031:222–228, 2005.
35. Lopresti BJ, Klunk WE, Mathis CA: Simplified quantification of Pittsburgh Compound β-amyloid imaging PET studies: a comparative analysis. J Nucl Med 46:1959–1972, 2005.

2

DEMENTIA

*Epidemiological Considerations, Nomenclature,
and a Tacit Consensus Definition*

John C. S. Breitner, M.D., M.P.H.

Epidemiological research addresses the distribution of disease in populations and the association of disease symptoms with identifiable factors that can provide clues to etiology or prevention. For dementia or any other condition, the ultimate objective of such research is the prevention of the disease or the mitigation of its consequences.

What Is a Case?

This is the first question for any epidemiological research. The definition of a case is a precondition to answering such other questions as secular changes in rates of disease occurrence, differences in geographic distribution, or association of the disease with risk or protective factors.

Amazingly, 50 years after the start of modern dementia research, our field lacks clarity on this fundamental question of definition. And yet we have achieved reasonable consensus about dementia incidence and prevalence and their change over

This chapter is reprinted from Breitner JCS: "Dementia—Epidemiological Considerations, Nomenclature, and a Tacit Consensus Definition." *Journal of Geriatric Psychiatry and Neurology* 19:129–136, 2006. Used with permission.

time. Almost certainly, this consensus has been possible only because experts in practice or research tacitly embrace a clinical concept of dementia, no matter what formal diagnostic criteria they espouse: *Diagnostic and Statistical Manual of Mental Disorders,* 3rd Edition (DSM-III), 3rd Edition, Revised (DSM-III-R), and 4th Edition (DSM-IV); and the *International Classification of Diseases*, 9th Revision (ICD-9) and 10th Revision (ICD-10); and so on. As a preamble to the description of some notable findings on the epidemiology of dementia, I therefore offer a digression on the concept of dementia that has been implicit but has been used almost universally de facto.

How It All Began

"Modern" dementia research began with the work of Martin Roth and colleagues in the 1950s. Roth challenged the then-prevailing concept of a unitary "senile psychosis," noting that some older hospitalized psychiatric patients had predominantly cognitive symptoms, whereas others suffered primarily from mood disorders, hallucinations, or delusions.[1] Roth used the term *dementia* (then rarely used) to describe the former group's condition, arguing that the patients suffered predominantly from "organic" illnesses of the brain, including neurodegenerative disorders and strokes. To emphasize the difference in prognosis in these patients compared with other elderly patients, he showed that the mortality in patients with dementia was increased.[2] The following decade yielded firm evidence that most instances of dementia reflected the presence of "organic" brain disease.[3–5] Notably, however, a diagnosis of these cases was always made before death on *clinical* grounds.

In one sense, Roth's seminal work may have done our field a disservice. His attempt to validate the distinction of dementing illness from other disorders by emphasizing their association with "organic" brain pathology was conflated over time to the view that they were one and the same. In adopting this perspective, Roth followed the then-current practice of diagnosing a clinical condition by its presumed etiology—a method that has long been abandoned elsewhere in psychiatry. Recall, for example, that the American Psychiatric Association's first *Diagnostic and Statistical Manual* (DSM) implied that every psychiatric diagnosis was "reaction" to a presumed cause (e.g., schizophrenic reaction, manic-depressive reaction). Roth's reasoning about dementia was less primitive than others, and, to his enormous credit, he fostered empirical investigation of his presumption that dementia was attributable to "organic" brain disease. But, to this writer at least, his seminal contribution was actually the identification of a clinical syndrome based on its constituent features.

So, What Is a Case?

The identification of clinical conditions based on distinctions in the phenomena of their presentation was a tradition of continental psychiatry, and particularly the work of Karl Jaspers.[6] Such a "phenomenological" approach to mental disorders in general, and to disorders of aging in particular, was promoted by Aubrey Lewis and his student Paul McHugh and by the latter's student Marshal Folstein. Folstein and McHugh argued that dementia was better defined exclusively as a clinical syndrome—the very syndrome that had enabled Roth to make the clinical distinction during his life between his patients with dementia and others.[7] For 40 years, McHugh and Folstein have taught the following simple definition of dementia: *Dementia is the clinical syndrome of mental life characterized by substantial global decline in cognitive function that is not attributable to alteration in consciousness.*

This definition works amazingly well, and nearly every one of its words is salient. Dementia is a *clinical syndrome,* meaning a constellation of signs and symptoms that, although recognizable in itself, may be attributable to numerous causes or pathological events. In this way, dementia is similar to such other useful medical syndromes as congestive heart failure, the nephrotic syndrome, or Cushing's syndrome. In contrast to these, however, dementia is a syndrome *of mental life.* The word *substantial* implies that the severity of the syndrome must be sufficient to cause impairment in daily function. The term *cognitive function* means simply that the principal changes in dementia are observed in the realm of cognition and not, for example, in mood, ideation, or perception. The word *global* means that several domains of cognition are affected, thus differentiating dementia from monofocal amnesia (Korsakoff's syndrome), aphasia, or other isolated abnormalities. *Decline* implies that the cognitive deficiency represents deterioration from a previous level of ability, thus distinguishing dementia from mental retardation or failure of intellectual development. Finally, the cognitive symptoms of dementia cannot be attributed to *alteration in consciousness,* which is the cardinal feature of delirium (in which cognition is also commonly affected).

Roth himself would probably not have disputed this definition of the *clinical syndrome* of dementia. But Roth advocated the principle that the core feature of dementia is the "organic" brain disease that is its cause. This principle encountered problems early, and they continue today. For example, if dementia is to be defined as "the clinical syndrome attributable to organic brain disease," then how do we classify patients whose clinical and pathological exams show that they have "dementia lacking distinctive histopathology"?[8] Roth's definition renders this term self-contradictory. More commonly, patients may have severe cognitive decline as a concomitant feature of geriatric depression, and this observation led Leslie Kiloh to coin the term "pseudo-dementia" to describe their condition—as distinguished from "true loss of intellectual capacity linked to irreversible brain disorder."[9]

Disagreement over exactly what was meant by "dementia" resulted in the following lively discussion between Roth and McHugh following a presentation of the latter's paper on the "Dementia Syndrome in Depression."[10]

> *Roth:* With the greatest friendliness, I should like to say to Dr. McHugh that I couldn't disagree with him less....If we had proceeded with his kind of classification

...and taken depressive dementia into the depressions, those distinctions I showed in life expectation and...outcome would have been completely blurred....It is rather like the medieval belief that all disease was a scourge of God, and therefore they were all one—you didn't have to make differences in prognosis. [And further,] Dementia carries the implication, the presumption of progression.

McHugh: Do you agree, Dr. Roth, that there are a certain number of affective disordered patients...who, when they are elderly have, with an attack of affective illness, a period of cognitive disability?

Roth: Yes, we are agreed that that happens, but that doesn't make them demented.

Clearly, these two distinguished academics were arguing at cross-purposes because of their different definitions of *dementia,* one syndromic and the other an appeal to a presumed etiology. Roth's comment that "dementia carries the implication, the presumption of progression" serves only to emphasize further the contrast between these approaches. What is a case, indeed?

Evolution of the Diagnostic Nomenclature

The Roth–McHugh debate occurred in 1976, but as one reviews successive revisions of DSM and ICD, it is clear that our field remains divided to this day on its core definition of dementia. Among the various sets of operational criteria for dementia, that of DSM-III appears most concordant with the Jaspers–Lewis–McHugh–Folstein definition. To review, the principal DSM-III criteria for dementia are as follows:

1. A loss of intellectual abilities of sufficient severity to interfere with social or occupational functioning;
2. Memory impairment; and
3. At least one of the following:
   a. Impairment of abstract thinking
   b. Impaired judgment
   c. Other disturbances of higher cortical function such as aphasia, apraxia, agnosia, or constructional difficulty
   d. Personality change
4. Change not attributable to alteration in consciousness.

Up to this point, these criteria are syndromic—that is, they do not suggest any specific cause. They also capture the key concept of decline ("loss"). The global aspect of dementia is captured by the need for impairment in memory as well as any of several other domains of cognitive ability. But DSM-III goes on to require

5. Evidence from history, physical examination, or laboratory of a specific etiological factor; or in the absence of such evidence, the presumption of such a factor.

Here one might reasonably ask, in what other field of practice does one base a definition on a presumption? But DSM-III also seems deficient in another respect. It insists on memory loss as part of the cognitive deficit. Although memory is commonly affected in those with global cognitive decline, this is not always the case (e.g., in frontotemporal dementia [FTD]).[11] As a result, strict DSM-III criteria do not classify many patients with FTD as having dementia. That hardly seems satisfactory.

The DSM-III-R revision did not help. In a subtle change, the word *loss* now disappears in favor of *impairment* of cognition. Thus, the essential concept of decline has disappeared. Furthermore, the insistence on memory loss seems to have been made worse, not better, by the new requirement for impairment in both short- and long-term memory (FTD patients rarely have any appreciable long-term memory loss until their condition is well advanced). Otherwise, little is changed from DSM-III.

Even more discouraging was the evolution to DSM-IV. That volume's section on dementia offers a text discussion of the syndrome and its common causes. Thus, "the disorders in the 'Dementia' section are characterized by the development of multiple cognitive deficits (including memory impairment)." But it does not offer any explicit set of operational criteria for the diagnosis of dementia. Instead, there are individual criteria for the diseases that commonly provoke dementia. Each such set of criteria begins with the same set of criteria for syndromic dementia, and these are the criteria that are typically implied when one speaks of "DSM-IV criteria for dementia," because, in reality, such criteria do not exist. The implied DSM-IV criteria are similar to those of DSM-III, but the text section explains that the cognitive deficits of the dementia syndrome "are due to the direct physiological effects of a general medical condition, to the persisting effects of a substance, or to multiple etiologies." One might wonder what is meant here by "general medical condition"— is Alzheimer's disease (AD) such a condition? Is this phrase meant to imply a DSM-III-like obeisance to Roth-style organicity? One may again question whether such vague language has a place in any definition.

Finally, with some misgiving, I suggest that the ICD-10 definition of dementia is the worst offender of all in confusing syndromic with etiologic reasoning. Here, dementia is categorized as part of a group of "organic mental disorders" that are "grouped together on the basis of their having in common a demonstrable etiology in cerebral disease, brain injury, or other insult leading to cerebral dysfunction." "Dementia," the ICD continues, "is a syndrome due to disease of the brain, usually of a chronic or progressive nature, in which there is disturbance of multiple higher cortical functions, including [it is not clear whether these are required] memory, thinking, orientation, comprehension, calculation, learning capacity, language, and judgement." This is vintage Roth.

Consequences of Confusion— Real and Imagined

The consequences of the logical difficulties and inconsistencies of the various criteria for dementia were demonstrated in an important paper by Erkinjuntti et al.[12] These authors reviewed the set of 442 individuals with suspected dementia whose history and examination were evaluated by a consensus of experts in the Canadian Study of Health and Aging (CSHA).[13] Each case was reviewed for its *strict* conformity to criteria of DSM-IV, ICD-10, or CAMDEX for dementia. The results are shown in Figure 2–1.

Saved by Clinical Judgment?

The CSHA investigators stated that they used DSM-III-R criteria for dementia. As noted above, these are very similar to DSM-IV criteria. Yet, the figure shows that nearly half of the patients with dementia did not meet DSM-IV or any other set of criteria strictly applied. The "clinical consensus" of experts diagnosed dementia in 393 participants. However, strict application of the "DSM-IV criteria" found only 256 case participants, including 56 whom the experts did not characterize as having dementia. Why? My conversations with other epidemiological investigators suggest that we all use the various criteria to the extent that they meet our own clinical concepts of dementia. Thus, for example, the Cache County Study used DSM-III-R criteria (ignoring the required presumption of etiology) but acknowledged that cases would be counted regardless of demonstrable deficits in *both* long- and short-term memory.[14] Figure 2–1 suggests that without such makeshift adjustments, it would not have been possible for the many studies in the United States, Europe, and indeed around the world to have found consistent incidence figures.

An Implied Definition Made Explicit

Here is a suggested formulation of the syndrome used tacitly by both clinicians and clinical epidemiologists. Because of its simplicity and practical utility, the following may also commend itself to psychiatrists more broadly.

1. The dementia syndrome involves a global deficit in cognitive abilities—that is, in several domains of cognitive activity. The global characteristic differentiates dementia from other cognitive syndromes in which a single cognitive domain is deficient (e.g., isolated amnestic disorder). Impairment of memory is typical in dementia but is not necessary to its definition. Other cognitive abilities that are frequently impaired include language functions (aphasia), ability to coordinate

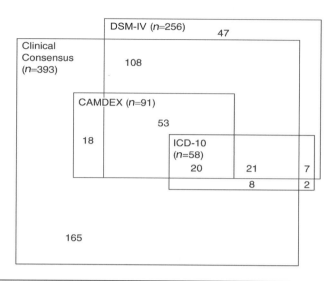

FIGURE 2–1. Patients identified as having dementia according to various diagnostic classification systems.

A total of 1,879 patients were evaluated. One patient in whom dementia was diagnosed according to DSM-IV and CAMDEX is not shown. DSM-IV = *Diagnostic and Statistical Manual of Mental Disorders*, 4th Edition; ICD-10 = *International Classification of Diseases*, 10th Revision.

and sequence ideas or movements (apraxia), and ability to recognize correctly objects that have been adequately perceived (agnosia). Deficits of abilities in reasoning, judgment, calculation, or so-called executive functioning are also common. Other behavioral, ideational, or perceptual disorders occur variably (e.g., agitation or aggression, delusions or overvalued ideas, hallucinations or illusions). Although the last mentioned are not a defining feature, they can complicate dementia, adding significantly to the burden or difficulty of its care.

2. The deficit represents a state of decline from a previously established level of abilities. Dementia is thus differentiated from syndromes that result from the failure of development of adequate cognitive or intellectual abilities. The decline is usually evident directly but can also be inferred from an educational, social, or occupational history that implies substantially better premorbid functional abilities.

3. The cognitive deficits or associated features are of sufficient severity to impair accustomed social or occupational functions.

4. The decline in cognition or functional abilities is not attributable to alteration in level of consciousness. In this way, dementia may be differentiated from delirium, another syndrome in which impaired cognition and behavioral or perceptual disturbance are common.

TABLE 2–1.   Prevalence rates observed for nine studies combined (with confidence interval) and estimates derived from fitted modified logistic model and from original exponential model

Age	N	Prevalence observed (%)	On modified logistic model	On original exponential model
65–69	1,459	1.53 (1.16–2.60)	1.50	1.30
70–74	4,740	3.54 (3.01–4.07)	3.54	2.43
75–79	6,291	6.80 (6.18–7.42)	7.30	4.45
80–84	4,327	13.57 (12.54–14.58)	13.40	8.14
85–89	4,191	22.26 (21.00–23.52)	22.17	14.91
90–94	1,388	31.48 (29.04–33.92)	33.00	27.31
95–99	317	44.48 (36.28–52.68)	44.80	50.20

Source.   Ritchie and Kildea.[16]

Resulting Progress in Dementia Epidemiology

Probably through recourse to the above tacit definition, our field appears to have produced reasonably consistent estimates for incidence rates by age.[15] Even comparisons of dementia prevalence are consistent—remarkably, because prevalence is a function of both incidence and survivorship of cases, and survivorship must vary widely over time and in different health systems and cultures. Table 2–1 and Figure 2–2 show results of an authoritative international meta-analysis of dementia presence in the developed world.[16]

Table 2–1 suggests a typical dementia prevalence of 10% at age 80, rising to 30% at age 90, and 45%–50% at age 95 and older. It bears mention that these are point prevalence figures and are not cumulative to a given age. The latter may be estimated as the definite integral of a parametric equation that describes the incidence of dementia as a function of age (see below).

As Table 2–2 suggests, the increase in incidence of moderate to severe dementia appears to be approximately exponential with age, doubling about every 5 years. Some key points to note from this table are that 1) the incidence of moderate to severe dementia is about 1% between ages 75 and 79; 2) the incidence of moderate to severe AD is about 1% at age 80; 3) in European studies, at least, the rates are some threefold higher for "mild" dementia and AD; and 4) after age 75, an ever-increasing proportion of all dementia is AD.

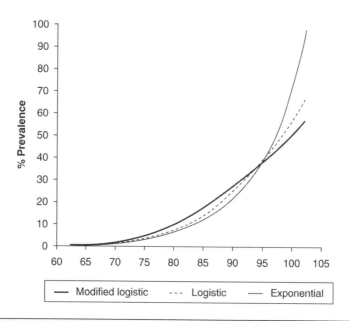

FIGURE 2–2.   Relation, expressed in three ways (modified logistic, logistic, and exponential), between age and prevalence of dementia in a meta-analysis of nine studies.

Source.   Ritchie and Kildea.[16]

Implications for Public Health

A quantitative review of the incidence literature[17] suggested a "best fit" exponential equation describing the relation of dementia incidence and age as follows:

$$\text{Incidence (\% per year)} = 0.084\,e^{0.142(t-60)}$$

where t = age.

The staggering public health implications of AD are well revealed by the fact that the cumulative incidence of AD, as estimated by integration of the above equation between ages 60 and 95 years, is 84%. This result is corroborated by recent findings from the Cache County Study, which found that 70%–75% of individuals would develop dementia by age 100, but with the comment that this figure was likely an underestimate attributable to the imperfect sensitivity of screening methods.[18]

These last observations raise concerns that the brain aging process we call AD is universal among humankind, with only the rate of its expression and the timing (age) of dementia occurrence differing among individuals. If so, then all "risk factors"

TABLE 2–2.   Meta-analytic estimates for incidence of dementia and Alzheimer's disease from the United States, Europe, and East Asia

| | Dementia | | | | Alzheimer's disease | | | |
| | Mild+ | | Moderate+ | | Mild+ | | Moderate+ | |
Age group (y)	Incidence	95% CI	Incidence	95% CI	Incidence	95% CI	Incidence	95% CI
Europe								
65–69	9.1	6.5–12.7	3.6	1.3–9.6	2.5	1.6–3.9	1.0	0.4–2.6
70–74	17.6	14.2–21.9	6.4	3.3–12.5	5.2	3.8–7.1	2.2	1.2–4.1
75–79	33.3	29.0–38.3	11.7	7.1–19.2	10.7	8.4–13.6	4.8	3.0–7.5
80–84	59.9	52.8–67.9	21.5	12.8–36.2	22.1	18.2–26.9	10.6	6.8–16.6
85–89	104.1	84.6–128.2	37.7	17.1–83.0	46.1	35.2–60.5	22.6	11.6–44.3
90–94	179.8	129.3–250.1	66.1	19.3–226.4	96.6	62.2–149.9	47.7	16.6–137.4
United States								
65–69			2.4	1.9–3.0	6.1	3.7–10.0	1.6	1.3–2.0
70–74			5.0	4.3–5.7	11.1	8.2–14.9	3.5	3.1–4.1
75–79			10.5	9.4–11.6	20.1	15.6–25.8	7.8	7.1–8.7
80–84			17.7	16.1–19.4	38.4	28.7–51.4	14.8	13.5–16.2
85–89			27.5	23.7–32.0	74.5	45.9–120.9	26.0	22.5–30.0

TABLE 2–2. Meta-analytic estimates for incidence of dementia and Alzheimer's disease from the United States, Europe, and East Asia *(continued)*

| | Dementia | | | | Alzheimer's disease | | | |
| | Mild+ | | Moderate+ | | Mild+ | | Moderate+ | |
Age group (y)	Incidence	95% CI	Incidence	95% CI	Incidence	95% CI	Incidence	95% CI
East Asia								
65–69	3.5	1.7–7.2			0.7	0.1–5.7		
70–74	7.1	4.6–11.1			2.1	0.6–7.0		
75–79	14.7	10.5–20.6			5.8	2.8–11.8		
80–84	32.6	24.8–42.9			14.9	9.4–23.7		
85–89	72.1	48.0–108.2			39.7	21.2–74.3		

Note.   CI=confidence interval.
Source.   Adapted from Jorm and Jolley.[15]

for AD must necessarily act as modifiers of the timing of disease expression. This timing effect has been shown most clearly for the genetic risk factor *APOE* ε4, which has been shown in one clinical sample and two epidemiological analyses to bear on the timing of disease onset but not on the number who will develop disease if they live to age 100.[18–20] Indeed, no known risk factor for AD has been shown to operate other than as a modifier of timing of onset.

Do the Rates Change Over Time?

If AD is a near-universal consequence of aging, the implication must be that, absent strong change in risk factor profiles over time, its age-specific incidence rates should not vary over time more than can be accounted for by methodological advances in case detection. The scant available evidence suggests that incidence rates have changed little if at all over the past three decades. At least one study attempted to use uniform diagnostic methods while reviewing three decades of records from residents of Olmsted County, almost all of whom received their health care at the Mayo Clinic.[21] Notwithstanding some methodological limitations from diagnoses assigned by chart review, this study suggested little or no change in age-specific incidence of dementia over three decenniums.

Sex Differences After Age 80

Several large studies now show that after age 80 or 85, the incidences of dementia and AD are substantially higher for women than for men.[22,23] Earlier studies reported roughly equivalent rates for men and women, but these studies typically investigated few individuals older than 80, which they collapsed into a single group. Because women tend to live longer than men, the more recent findings again have ominous public health implications.

Does Alzheimer's Disease Incidence Decline in Extreme Old Age?

A number of studies suggest that the incidence of dementia may no longer increase, but may in fact decrease, at ages after the mid-90s.[22,24] If true, these findings could reflect a phenomenon of variable susceptibility in which the most vulnerable at-risk elements of the population become depleted because all have developed dementia, leaving only a small residue of relatively less susceptible people. Two methodological advances are needed to investigate this finding further. First, it would be extremely desirable to obtain substantial numbers of brain autopsies from survivors in their late 90s or older. Do they have AD pathology without dementia? We know this happens, but we do not know how often, especially at such late ages. Second, we need improved methods of dementia diagnosis in extreme old age. Only now are the major AD centers seeing substantial numbers of very old people, so perhaps this problem will resolve itself. Still, for this purpose, it would probably make sense for the AD program of the National Institute on Aging to encourage recruitment of very old people into its Alzheimer's Disease Research Centers and Core Centers.

Differences in Incidence by Geographic Region and Their Implications

Finally, we may review some data on regional differences in dementia occurrence. Like the secular trend issue, this is a difficult question to resolve because of methodological problems. Over the past decade, however, one study group has successfully compared dementia rates in the Yoruba people of Ibadan, Nigeria, versus those of African Americans (mostly of West African descent) in Indianapolis, Indiana.[25]

Figure 2–3 shows the findings for dementia and for AD. The two parts of the figure also compare the rates of these two populations with rates found in other widely cited incidence studies. The figure suggests, first, that the Ibadan and Indianapolis rates for dementia and AD are near the upper and lower bounds, respectively, for representative rates from other surveys. Second, the rates in Indianapolis appear to be approximately threefold higher than those from Ibadan. Although the assumption of identical gene pools for the two populations is approximate at best, these results still provide strong evidence that environmental factors—for example, diet (and correlated hypertensive or arteriosclerotic cardiovascular and cerebrovascular disease)—bear strongly on the age-specific risk of dementia.

Evaluation of Genetic and Environmental Risks

Twin studies are not generally used for identification of individual genetic traits or environmental influences, but population-based twin research can provide important estimates of the genetic and environmental contribution to phenotypic variation. Two recent studies from the Swedish Twin Registry have provided important information on this topic.[26,27] Along with other studies,[28] the Swedish research shows no evidence of shared environmental influence (similarities within sibships that are not attributable to genes), but it estimates unique (unshared, typically adult) environmental influence at 20%–35%, with the remaining 65%–80% of variation in AD susceptibility attributable to genes. The genetic influence does not appear to wane substantially with age, at least through age 85.[27]

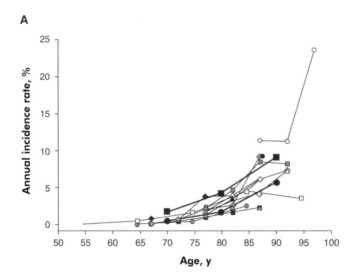

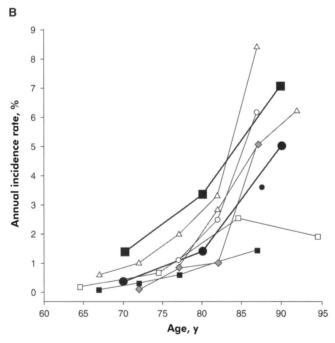

FIGURE 2–3.   Annual incidence rates of dementia (A) and Alzheimer's disease (B).

Rates for African Yoruba (Ibadan) in dark circles versus African Americans (Indianapolis) in dark squares.

Along with the Indianapolis–Ibadan data, the Swedish estimates of a 20%–35% environmental contribution emphasize the potential of environmental risk factor modification for the prevention of AD. To interpret these percentages, one must recall that heritability and environmentality are *proportions* of the contribution to phenotypic variance. Because AD has very strong genetic risk factors, a 20%–35% contribution of the environment is substantial. Apart from very rare mutations that cause early-onset AD, there are no securely identified "AD genes" except for the *APOE* polymorphism. The *APOE* locus accounts for something like 40% of the population attributable risk (PAR) for AD.[29,30] Although PAR is not identical to heritability, it is conceptually related, so that it is likely that *APOE* accounts for about half the total genetic contribution to AD, with the remaining half still awaiting secure identification of other genes. The implication is that adult environmental influences probably account for about half the variation of risk attributable to *APOE*. Because a single *APOE* ε4 allele accelerates onset of AD by some 10 years, the environment may account for about 5 years' variation in onset. Much more work is needed to find the individual risk factors that create this variation and to develop interventions based on those findings.

Summary and Conclusion

Despite differences in specific diagnostic criteria, the dementia syndrome has achieved widespread and relatively uniform recognition by clinicians and researchers alike. Our tacit recognition of this syndrome has enabled considerable advance in the difficult field of dementia epidemiology. The syndrome now deserves a formal statement of definition. Although dementia is recognized as being consequent in most instances to structural or neurodegenerative alteration in the brain, this is not a defining feature. It is an important goal in dementia research, as in all of medicine, that we characterize the underlying pathological or etiologic entity responsible for the clinical picture. However, that pursuit is consequent to the reliable recognition of the dementia syndrome itself: first things first. Only by proceeding in this orderly and logical fashion will we be in the strongest position for future advances.

References

1.	Roth M, Morrissey JD: Problems in the diagnosis and classification of mental disorder in old age, with a study of case material. J Ment Sci 98:66–80, 1952.
2.	Roth M: The natural history of mental disorder in old age. J Ment Sci 101:281?301, 1955.
3.	Corsellis JAN: Mental Illness and the Ageing Brain (Maudsley Monogr No 9). London, Oxford University Press, 1962.

4. Tomlinson BE, Blessed G, Roth M: Observations on the brains of demented old people. J Neurol Sci 11:205–242, 1970.

5. Tomlinson BE, Blessed G, Roth M: Observations on the brains of non-demented old people. J Neurol Sci 7:331–356, 1968.

6. Jaspers K: General Psychopathology, Vols 1 and 2. Baltimore, MD, Johns Hopkins University Press, 1997.

7. McHugh PR, Slavney PR: The Perspectives of Psychiatry, 2nd Edition. Baltimore, MD, Johns Hopkins University Press, 1998.

8. Giannakopoulos P, Hof PR, Bouras C: Dementia lacking distinctive histopathology: clinicopathological evaluation of 32 cases. Acta Neuropathol (Berl) 89:346–355, 1996.

9. Kiloh LG: Pseudo-dementia. Acta Psychiatr Scand 37:336–351, 1961.

10. McHugh P, Folstein MF: Dementia syndrome in depression, in Aging, Vol 7. Edited by Katzman R, Terry RD, Bick K. New York, Raven, 1977, pp 94–96.

11. Neary D, Snowden J, Mann D: Frontotemporal dementia. Lancet Neurol 4:771–780, 2005.

12. Erkinjuntti T, Ostbye T, Steenhuis R, et al: The effect of different diagnostic criteria on the prevalence of dementia. N Engl J Med 333:1667–1674, 1997.

13. Rockwood K, Stadnyk K: The prevalence of dementia in the elderly: a review. Can J Psychiatry 39:253–257, 1994.

14. Breitner J, Wyse B, Anthony JC, et al: APOE-ε4 count predicts age when prevalence of AD increases, then declines. The Cache County Study. Neurology 53:321–331, 1999.

15. Jorm AF, Jolley D: The incidence of dementia: a meta-analysis. Neurology 51:728–733, 1998.

16. Ritchie K, Kildea D: Is senile dementia "age-related" or "ageing-related"?—evidence from meta-analysis of dementia prevalence in the oldest old. Lancet 346:931–934, 1995.

17. Brookmeyer R, Gray S, Kawas C: Projections of Alzheimer's disease in the United States and the public health impact of delaying disease onset. Am J Public Health 88:1337–1342, 1998.

18. Khachaturian A, Corcoran C, Mayer L, et al: Apolipoprotein E ε4 count affects age at onset of Alzheimer's disease but not lifetime susceptibility. The Cache County Study. Arch Gen Psychiatry 61:518–524, 2004.

19. Corder E, Saunders A, Strittmatter W: Gene dose of apolipoprotein E type 4 allele and the risk of Alzheimer's disease in late onset families. Science 261:921–923, 1993.

20. Meyer M, Tschanz J, Norton M, et al: APOE genotype predicts when—not whether—one is predisposed to develop Alzheimer disease. Nat Genet 19:321–322, 1998.

21. Kokmen E, Beard CM, O'Brien P, et al: Is the incidence of dementing illness changing? A 25-year time trend study in Rochester, Minnesota (1960–1984). Neurology 43:1887–1892, 1993.

22. Fratiglioni L, Launer LJ, Andersen K, et al: Incidence of dementia and major subtypes in Europe: a collaborative study of population-based cohorts. Neurologic Diseases in the Elderly Research Group. Neurology 54 (11, suppl 5):S10–S15, 2000.

23. Zandi PP, Carlson MC, Plassman BL, et al, Cache County Memory Study Investigators: Hormone replacement therapy and incidence of Alzheimer disease in older women: the Cache County Study. JAMA 288:2123–2129, 2002.

24. Miech RA, Breitner JC, Zandi PP, et al: Incidence of AD may decline in the early 90s for men, later for women: The Cache County study. Neurology 58:209–218, 2002.

25. Hendrie HC, Ogunniyi A, Hall KS, et al: Incidence of dementia and Alzheimer disease in 2 communities: Yoruba residing in Ibadan, Nigeria, and African Americans residing in Indianapolis, Indiana. JAMA 285:739–747, 2001.

26. Gatz M, Reynolds CA, Fratiglioni L, et al: Role of genes and environments for explaining Alzheimer disease. Arch Gen Psychiatry 63:168–174, 2006.

27. Pedersen NL, Gatz M, Berg S, et al: How heritable is Alzheimer's disease late in life? Findings from Swedish twins. Ann Neurol 55:180–185, 2004.

28. Meyer JM, Breitner JC: Multiple threshold model for the onset of Alzheimer's disease in the NAS-NRC twin panel. Am J Med Genet 81:92–97, 1998.

29. Ashford JW: APOE genotype effects on Alzheimer's disease onset and epidemiology. J Mol Neurosci 23:157–165, 2004.

30. Slooter AJ, Cruts M, Kalmijn S, et al: Risk estimates of dementia by apolipoprotein E genotypes from a population-based incidence study: the Rotterdam Study. Arch Neurol 55:964–968, 1998.

3

DIAGNOSTIC CRITERIA IN DEMENTIA

A Comparison of Current Criteria, Research Challenges, and Implications for DSM-V and ICD-11

Barry Reisberg, M.D.
Norman Sartorius, M.D., Ph.D.

Dr. Reisberg's research has been supported in part by U.S. Department of Health and Human Services (DHHS) grants AG 03051, AG 08051, 09127, and AG 11505, from the National Institute on Aging of the National Institutes of Health (NIH); by grants 90AZ 2791, 90AM 2552, and 90AR 2160 from the DHHS Administration on Aging; by grant NCRR M01 RR00096 from the General Clinical Research Center Program of the National Center for Disease Research Resources of the NIH; by the Fisher Center for Alzheimer's Disease Research Foundation; and by grants from Mr. William Silberstein and Mr. Leonard Litwin.

This chapter is adapted from Reisberg B: "Diagnostic Criteria in Dementia: A Comparison of Current Criteria." *Journal of Geriatric Psychiatry and Neurology* 19:137–146, 2006. Used with permission.

Current diagnostic criteria in dementia are embodied in the American Psychiatric Association's *Diagnostic and Statistical Manual of Mental Disorders*, 4th Edition, Text Revision (DSM-IV-TR),[1] published in the year 2000, and the World Health Organization's *International Classification of Diseases,* 10th Revision (ICD-10),[2] published in 1992. Review of these current diagnostic manuals reveals many strengths, and some weaknesses, from the perspective of present advances in scientific knowledge and associated nosological consensus. This brief critique will contrast these current criteria from the present perspective and identify suggested revisions as well as research directions that might optimize DSM-V and ICD-11 descriptions.

Overall Rubric of the Dementias

DSM-IV-TR classifies dementias within the framework termed "delirium, dementia, and amnestic and other cognitive disorders." The ICD-10 classifies these conditions within the framework of "organic, including symptomatic, mental disorders (F00–F09)."

DSM-IV-TR contains a critique of the ICD-10 diagnostic rubric. It states, "The term *organic mental disorder* is no longer used in DSM-IV because it incorrectly implies that 'nonorganic' mental disorders do not have a biological basis."[1(p.135)] In DSM-IV-TR, this critique applies to the prior DSM-III-R categorization of "organic mental syndromes and disorders." However, irrespective of the focus of this critique, it is becoming increasingly clear to all investigators and practitioners that the DSM-IV-TR critique is meritorious. Biological bases for, concomitants of, and elements in all mental disorders are increasingly being identified. There is no longer any viable rationale for the *organic/nonorganic* dichotomy, and it should be abandoned.

With respect to the DSM-IV-TR classification of "delirium, dementia, and amnestic and other cognitive disorders," it is suggested herein that the more parsimonious terminology "cognitive disorders" might be most suitable for this category. Nothing is lost by using the more compact description, and the concept is more readily conveyed.

DEMENTIA

Both DSM-IV-TR and the ICD-10 have categories termed "dementia," although this category is much more clearly delineated in DSM-IV-R than in ICD-10. In DSM-IV-TR, it is noted that "a dementia is categorized by multiple cognitive deficits that include impairment in memory."[1(p.135)] ICD-10 defines dementia as "a syndrome due to disease of the brain, usually of a chronic or progressive nature, in which there is disturbance of multiple higher cortical functions, including memory, thinking, orientation, comprehension, calculation, learning capacity, language, and judgement. Consciousness is not clouded. The impairments of cognitive functions are commonly accompanied, and occasionally preceded, by deterioration in emotional control, social behavior or motivation."

There are three major critiques of the brief DSM-IV-TR definition of dementia. These are as follows. First, the DSM-IV-TR definition of dementia does not specify that these are acquired conditions. Hence, the amentias attributable to perinatal conditions, mental subnormalities that become manifest in childhood, and so forth are not differentiated and indeed would appear to fall within the DSM-IV-TR dementia definition.

Second, the DSM-IV-TR definition of dementia necessitates "impairment in memory." This criterion is contrary to consensus definitions and clinical experience with many dementia disorders. For example, prominent dementing diseases such as vascular dementia and frontotemporal dementia (FTD) are characteristically not marked by impairment of memory. In the words of a recent consensus statement on vascular cognitive impairment and dementia, "memory impairment is not necessarily a prime symptom in vascular dementia."[3] Similarly, for FTD (sometimes termed frontotemporal lobar dementia [FTLD]), a consensus has noted that "the most common clinical manifestation of FTLD is...with relative preservation of memory function."[4] The most prominent FTD subtype is Pick's disease. Both ICD-10 and DSM-IV-TR have definitions of Pick's disease that either de-emphasize the occurrence of memory impairment or note its late occurrence in the evolution of the disorder. In the words of the ICD-10, dementia in Pick's disease (F02.0) is "a progressive dementia...characterized by early, slowly progressing changes of character and social deterioration, followed by impairment of intellect, memory and language functions." DSM-IV-TR also notes that "Pick's disease is characterized clinically by changes in personality early in the course, deterioration in social skills, emotional blunting, behavioral disinhibition, and prominent language abnormalities. Difficulties with memory, apraxia, and other features of dementia usually follow later in the course."[1(p.165)] Hence, by any criterion, including internal consistency as well as external validity, impairment in memory should not be a necessary criterion for a dementia diagnosis.

The third deficiency in the DSM-IV-TR definition of dementia is that it omits mention of functional (i.e., the ability to carry out activities) or behavioral/emotional changes. As already noted in the above discussion, with respect to, for example, FTD, these may be very prominent modalities of dementia presentation and course.

DSM-IV-TR elaborates on the definition of dementia noted above in the section on diagnostic features. It notes that "the essential feature of dementia is development of multiple cognitive deficits that include memory impairment and at least one of the following cognitive disturbances: aphasia, apraxia, agnosia, or a disturbance in executive functioning. The cognitive deficits must be sufficiently severe to cause impairment in occupational or social functioning and must represent a decline from a previously higher level of functioning."[1(p.148)]

The functional portion of the above definition is excellent. However, apart from the matter of memory impairment, already discussed, the prominence of early (diagnostic) deficits in aphasia, apraxia, and agnosia should be critiqued. Medical and lay definitions of these conditions from standard dictionaries are shown in Table 3–1. It will be noted from these definitions that these symptoms are most readily associated with brain trauma, frequently of acute origin. For example, aphasia, apraxia, and agnosia, as defined, would commonly be noted after brain injury or a stroke. If one takes the example of the most common form of dementia, Alzheimer's disease (AD), these symptoms do not become overtly evident until the latter portion of the disease. Of course, ultimately, with the advance of AD, virtually all cognitive and motoric capacities are lost.[7] In the words of DSM-IV-TR, in the description of "dementia of the Alzheimer's type" (294.1x), "A common pattern is...early deficits in recent memory followed by the development of aphasia, apraxia, and agnosia after several years."[1 (p.156)] Hence, it appears that a definition of dementia, with ultimate validity later in the process, when all cognitive capacities are overtly lost, is being superimposed on early diagnosis, probably on the basis of medical traditions from findings in brain trauma and stroke. The ICD-10 description of dementia as a "disturbance of multiple higher cortical functions, including memory, thinking, orientation, comprehension, calculation, learning capacity, language, and judgement," would appear to be far more descriptive of the nature of losses in dementia.

In summary, a critique of the DSM-IV-TR definition of dementia includes the following major points: 1) dementia is diverse, and memory deficit is not the only presentation of dementia; and 2) dementia is characterized by multiple cognitive deficits, functional deficits, and, commonly, behavioral/personality changes.

The ICD-10 definition of dementia is an excellent and accurate summary. However, some small improvements can be recommended. In sum, it is recommended that this definition be modified as shown in Table 3–2. These modifications include the following changes:

1. The term *cortical functions* is replaced by the term *cortical capacities,* because the word *functions* has multiple higher-order and specific meanings, even in this brief definition, and becomes ambiguous when used in these multiple definitional/conceptual contexts.
2. The word *generally* is introduced, because the multiple higher cortical capacity deficits are not necessarily all manifest, particularly early in the dementia process.
3. A statement regarding true functional deficits as concomitants of the dementia process is introduced. These include executive functioning deficits and, depending on severity, instrumental (complex) and basic activity of daily life (basic skills) deficits.
4. Finally, current knowledge regarding affective, motivational, and emotional changes; perceptual changes; and motoric and coordination changes with the evolution of dementia pathology is alluded to.[7]

TABLE 3–1. Definitions of aphasia, apraxia, and agnosia

	Standard lay definition[a]	Standard medical definition[b]
Aphasia	"The loss or impairment of the power to use words as symbols of ideas that results from a brain lesion"	"Any of a large group of speech disorders involving deficit or loss of the power of expression by speech, writing or signs, or of comprehending spoken or written language, due to or disease of the brain or to psychogenic causes. Less severe forms are known as dysphasias."
Apraxia	"Loss or impairment of ability to execute movements (as in manipulating objects) without muscular paralysis"	"Loss of ability to carry out familiar, purposeful movements in the absence of paralysis or other motor or sensory impairment"
Agnosia	"The potential or complete loss of the ability to recognize familiar objects by seeing, hearing, or touching and usu[ally] as a result of brain damage"	"Loss of the power to recognize the import of sensory stimuli"

[a]From *Webster's Third New International Dictionary,* Unabridged, 1993.[5]
[b]From *Dorland's Illustrated Medical Dictionary,* 2003.[6]

Alzheimer's Disease

This brief review acknowledges the many strengths in the current diagnostic criteria. Any future criteria will build on these strengths. However, there are also weaknesses from the perspective of current scientific knowledge. A few weaknesses in the criteria for AD that will need to be addressed in future diagnostic criteria are described herein.

DICHOTOMY OF ALZHEIMER'S DISEASE INTO EARLY AND LATE ONSET

The ICD-10 divides AD into 1) dementia in AD with early onset (F00.0) and 2) dementia in AD with late onset (F00.1).

Dementia in AD with early onset is defined as "with onset before the age of 65, with a relatively rapid deteriorating course and with marked multiple disorders

TABLE 3–2.   Dementia: suggested modified definition from the
International Classification of Diseases, 10th Revision (ICD-10)

Dementia is a syndrome due to disease of the brain, usually of a chronic or
progressive nature, in which there is disturbance of multiple higher cortical
[functions] *capacities,* generally including memory, thinking, orientation,
comprehension, calculation, learning capacity, language, and judgment.
Consciousness is not [clouded] *compromised. The impairments of cognitive
capacities are accompanied by deficits in executive functioning and, depending
on the severity of the condition, may be accompanied by numerous other
functional losses in complex and basic skills. The* cognitive and *functional
impairments* are commonly accompanied, and [occasionally] *sometimes*
preceded, by [deterioration] *affective changes, motivational changes, emotional
changes, perceptual changes, and motoric and coordinational changes.*

Note.   Deletions in ICD-10 (1992)[2] text are shown in brackets. Insertions are shown in
italics. The final sentence in the ICD-10 text definition (see also text of the ICD-10 for
the original ICD-10 definition) has been replaced by the final sentence in this table.

of the higher cortical functions." Dementia in AD with late onset is defined as "with
onset after the age of 65, usually in the late 70s or thereafter, with a slow progression, and with memory impairment as the principal feature."

DSM-IV-TR also divides dementia of the Alzheimer's type (294.1x) into two
subtypes that require specification: 1) *with early onset,* if the onset is at age 65 years
or below, and 2) *with late onset,* if the onset is after 65 years.

These dichotomies of AD into early and late onset in both the ICD-10 and
DSM-IV-TR are not supportable by current scientific evidence. Indeed, they have
probably been obsolete since 1974, with the appearance of a publication by Hachinski
et al.[8] declaring AD a major illness on the basis primarily of the findings of Roth et
al.,[9] Blessed et al.,[10] and Tomlinson et al.,[11,12] published between 1966 and 1970.

A brief outline of the history of AD is shown in Table 3–3. Plaques in the brain
had been related to the pathology of senile dementia prior to Alzheimer's 1907 description of a woman who exhibited symptoms of the illness that were first noted
at 51 years of age.[13–15] The illness lasted 4½ years, ending with the patient's de-
mise. Alzheimer performed an autopsy on this woman, finding the neurofibrillary
tangles as well as the plaques that had previously been described by Blocq and
Marinesco[13] and Redlich.[14] Emil Kraepelin named the new illness "Alzheimer's disease" after his departmental faculty member. However, Alzheimer set back concectu-
alizations of his eponymously named disease in certain ways, at the same time as
he advanced conceptualizations in other ways. Alzheimer believed that his disease
occurred exclusively before the age of 65. When senile dementia occurred after the
age of 65, Alzheimer believed that the neurofibrillary tangles (described originally
by him) and the plaques (described in senile dementia in 1898 by Redlich) did not

TABLE 3–3. Brief history of Alzheimer's disease

Plaques observed in the brain.	1892	Blocq and Marinesco[13]
Plaques related to the pathology of senile dementia.	1898	Redlich[14]
Neurofibrillary change described and related to the pathology of presenile dementia.	1907	Alzheimer[15]
Kraepelin names illness "Alzheimer's disease."		
Alzheimer believes plaques and neurofibrillary tangles do not occur after age 65 and senile dementia is caused by atherosclerosis.		
Senile plaques, neurofibrillary tangles, and granulovacuolar degeneration demonstrated in normal aging and senile dementia.	1927 1933	Grunthal[16] Gellerstedt[17]
Neurofibrillary change related to pathology of senile dementia.	1959 1962	Margolis[18] Hirano and Zimmerman[19]
Cerebral arteriosclerosis differentiated from senile dementia.	1965	Corsellis and Evans[20]
Correlation between senile plaques and senile dementia established.	1962 1966 1968	Corsellis[21] Roth et al.[9] Blessed et al.[10]
Senile dementia and presenile dementia demonstrated to be similar or identical entities.	1968 1970	Tomlinson et al.[11] Tomlinson et al.[12]
Alzheimer's disease proclaimed a major illness.	1974	Hachinski et al.[8]

occur. Alzheimer attributed dementia occurring after the age of 65 to arteriosclerosis. This misconception of Alzheimer, that his disease was strictly one of presenile onset, was challenged in subsequent decades, notably by Grunthal (1927)[16] and Gellerstedt (1933),[17] who found that Alzheimer was wrong in that plaques and neurofibrillary tangles occurred in the brains of normal aged persons and also in persons with senile (i.e., onset at ages over 65 years) dementia. In subsequent work, Margolis (1959)[18] and Hirano and Zimmerman (1962)[19] found that neurofibrillary change was related to the pathology of senile dementia. However, Alzheimer's concepts did not begin to be effectively challenged until the work of Corsellis and Evans (1965),[20] who failed to find a marked association between arteriosclerosis and senile dementia. Corsellis (1962)[21] and then Sir Martin Roth, Bernard Tomlinson, and Gary Blessed, in a series of publications,[9–12] demonstrated not only the occurrence of plaques and tangles in older persons with dementia, but also correlations between these pathologies and the magnitude of dementia. As a result of these findings, AD, previously considered a rare illness occurring exclusively before the age of 65, came to be recognized as a major illness and, indeed, the same illness as Alois Alzheimer had observed in the presenium. Scientists abandoned the presenile/senile dementia dichotomy for AD in the early 1980s. Nevertheless, the dichotomy appears to have remained in the diagnostic nomenclature literature, although not in the scientific literature.

The so-called late-life form of AD, with overtly diagnosable dementia pathology, is rarely observed before the age of 49. Subsequently, the occurrence increases with increasing age. The late-life form of AD has been associated with at least one inherited genetic risk factor—that is, the nature of the apolipoprotein E genotype allelic status (specifically, the number of copies of the apolipoprotein ε, ε2, ε3, and ε4 alleles). However, the late-life form of AD has not been associated with genetic mutations.

It is now known that there are also rare forms of AD that are associated with genetic mutations. Scores of such mutations have been identified. The three most common are presenilin 1 (PS1) and 2 (PS2) and amyloid precursor protein (APP) mutations. Together, the genetically determined forms of AD are believed to account for less than 1% of dementias. These mutations produce an AD onset at various ages depending on the specific mutation. A recent review noted that 144 mutations in PS1, 10 mutations in PS2, and 19 different AD-associated mutations in the APP have been identified[22] (see Alzheimer Disease & Frontotemporal Dementia Mutation database: http://www.molgen.ua.ac.be/ADmutations and the Alzheimer's Research Forum genetic database, "Alzgene": http://www.alzgene.org, for up-to-date information). Mean onset for specific mutations can be as early as the third decade of life. When an Alzheimer's-type dementia occurs after the age of approximately 48 years, it is likely attributable to classical "late-onset" AD. Hence, it is recommended that the presenile/senile dichotomy at age 65 in the ICD-10 and DSM-IV-TR be abandoned.

DEFINITIONS OF ALZHEIMER'S DISEASE

The ICD-10 defines "dementia in Alzheimer's disease" as follows: "Alzheimer's disease is a primary degenerative cerebral disease of unknown etiology with characteristic neuropathological and neurochemical features. The disorder is usually insidious in onset and develops slowly but steadily over a period of several years." This is an excellent definition in general. However, it omits the clinical features and course of the disease.

DSM-IV-TR, in defining "dementia of the Alzheimer's type," stipulates that "the diagnosis can be made only when other etiologies for the dementia have been ruled out." In terms of the course of the condition, DSM-IV-TR notes that "early deficits in recent memory [are] followed by the development of aphasia, apraxia and agnosia after several years."[1(p.156)] Both of these statements must be critiqued.

Although the ICD-10 uses the term *Alzheimer's disease,* DSM-IV-TR uses *dementia of the Alzheimer's type* and emphasizes that DAT is a diagnosis of exclusion. Interestingly, or perhaps disturbingly, AD is the only dementia entity in DSM-IV-TR that is a diagnosis of exclusion. It is also the only dementia for which the standard "dementia workup" is suggested. Indeed, not only is Alzheimer's disease the only dementia entity that is considered a diagnosis of exclusion, but it also may have a unique role as a specified diagnosis of exclusion among mental illnesses and indeed medical and mental illnesses more generally. For example, schizophrenia, affective disorders, anxiety disorders, substance use disorders, and personality disorders are not considered diagnoses of exclusion. Similarly, myocardial infarctions and other medical conditions are not generally referred to as diagnoses of exclusion. The reasons for this unique distinction for AD derive from the historic nature of its "discovery." The history of this discovery has already been summarized in this chapter. At the time of the discovery of the importance of AD, in the late 1970s, the clinical features of the illness were relatively unknown. Beginning, in the 1980s, with the burgeoning interest in AD, the clinical features were increasingly well described. However, at the time of the McKhann et al. (1984)[23] criteria, these clinical features were just emerging from the literature and only beginning to be recognized. Assessment of AD with mental status assessments and dementia tests such as the Mental Status Questionnaire,[24] the Mini-Mental State Examination (MMSE),[25] and the Blessed Dementia Test and Blessed Information, Memory, and Concentration Test,[26] and even with assessments designed for pharmacotherapeutic efficacy trials, such as the Sandoz Clinical Assessment—Geriatric scale,[27] was already widely practiced. However, none of these measures distinguished AD from dementia resulting from, for example, head trauma or tumor. These descriptions of the dementia of AD became increasingly detailed over the course of the 1980s and subsequently. Consensus conferences in the past decade have concluded that AD should no longer be considered a diagnosis of exclusion. One of these consensus conferences was sponsored by the International Psychogeriatric Association, with the cosponsorship of Alzheimer's Disease International, the European Federation of Neurological Societies, the World Health Organization, and the World Psychiatric Association. It concluded that "there is agreement that AD is a characteristic clinicopathological entity that is amenable to diagnosis. The diagnosis of AD should no longer be considered one of exclusion. Rather, the diagnostic process is one of recognition of the characteristic features of AD and of conditions that can have an impact on presentation or mimic aspects of the clinicopathological picture."[28] Another consensus statement from the American Association for Geriatric Psychiatry, the Alzheimer's Association, and the American Geriatrics Society has also concluded, "Although the diagnosis of AD is often missed or delayed, it is primarily one of inclusion, not exclusion, and usually can be made using standardized clinical criteria. Most cases can be diagnosed...in primary care settings, yet some patients...benefit from specialist referral."[29]

Apart from the matter of AD being a diagnosis of exclusion, the statements in DSM-IV-TR regarding the course of AD should also be critiqued in view of present knowledge. As mentioned previously, DSM-IV-TR notes that "early deficits in recent memory [are] followed by the development of aphasia, apraxia and agnosia after several years." This statement is probably the result of a purely "MMSE-centric" view of AD. The MMSE was designed to be a screening instrument for dementia pathology. It is well known that the MMSE is subject to ceiling and floor effects in AD.[30–32] The MMSE also samples numerous areas of dementia pathology with only 30 items.

Studies that have examined the development of dementia pathology in the course of AD have noted that deficits in numerous areas, when assessed sensitively, proceed in a concomitant manner.[33] For example, the MMSE assesses praxis ability by requiring the participant to copy two interlocking pentagons.[25] However, others have found that having a participant draw a cube is a very sensitive indicator of praxic deficit in comparison with the copying of interlocking pentagons.[33,34] When assessed with sensitive measures, praxic capacity is a sensitive indicator of early dementia in AD.[33,34] Similarly, the loss of language ability in AD occurs early and continuously from the perspective of, for example, Wechsler Adult Intelligence Scale vocabulary scores.[35,36] Future diagnostic criteria should reflect the actual clinical symptomatology of AD as it evolves from the mild to the most severe stages.

Vascular Dementia

ICD-10 defines the entity vascular dementia (F01) as follows: "Vascular dementia is the result of infarction of the brain due to vascular disease, including hypertensive cerebrovascular disease. The infarcts are usually small but cumulative in their effect. Onset is usually in later life." It is noted that this entity includes arteriosclerotic dementia. The ICD-10 lists subtypes of vascular dementia (Table 3–4).

DSM-IV-TR describes vascular dementia (290.4x) (formerly multi-infarct dementia) as follows: "There must be evidence of cerebrovascular disease (i.e., focal neurological signs and symptoms or laboratory evidence) that is judged to be etiologically related to the dementia. The focal neurological signs and symptoms include extensor plantar response, pseudobulbar palsy, gait abnormalities, exaggeration of deep tendon reflexes, or weakness of an extremity." Computed tomography and magnetic resonance imaging of the head "usually demonstrate multiple vascular lesions of the cerebral cortex and subcortical structures."

The DSM-IV-TR definition of vascular dementia requires critique in a few areas. Most important, although the previously used terminology of multi-infarct dementia is no longer used, the concept of multi-infarct dementia is adopted in the definition. This concept no longer fits the great majority of patients who might

TABLE 3–4. Vascular dementia: subtypes from the *International Classification of Diseases,* 10th Revision (ICD-10)

Vascular dementia of acute onset (F01.0)
Multi-infarct dementia (F01.1)
Subcortical vascular dementia (F01.2)
Mixed cortical and subcortical vascular dementia (F01.3)
Other vascular dementia (F01.8)
Vascular dementia, unspecified (F01.9)

presently fall within the rubric of vascular dementia. In addition, the definition of vascular dementia used does not explicitly acknowledge the neurologic symptoms that commonly occur with the evolution of dementia pathology in, for example, AD. However, the DSM-IV-TR definition of vascular dementia is not incorrect in that it does refer to focal neurologic signs and symptoms. With the evolution of dementia pathology in AD, patients develop extensor plantar responses, gait abnormalities, and exaggerated deep tendon reflexes, as well other neurologic signs and symptoms.[37,38] Although there is a tendency for these symptoms to become manifest bilaterally, varying degrees of asymmetry occur. Therefore, in the current definitional context, it is suggested that the words "generally unilateral" deficits be added for the concept of infarct-related dementia. Also, common neurologic signs and symptoms in AD and other noninfarct dementias might be explicitly acknowledged.

In terms of the infarct concept for vascular dementia, DSM-IV-TR notes in associated findings that "a single stroke may cause a relatively circumscribed change in mental state…but generally does not cause Vascular Dementia, which typically results from the occurrence of multiple strokes, usually at different times." The age at onset is described as "typically earlier than that of Dementia of the Alzheimer's Type." The prevalence is described as "much less common than" that of DAT.

A recent consensus on vascular cognitive impairment concluded that "the current narrow definition of vascular dementia should be broadened to recognize the important part cerebrovascular disease plays in several cognitive disorders, including the hereditary vascular dementias, multi-infarct dementia, post stroke dementia, subcortical ischemic vascular disease and dementia, mild cognitive impairment and degenerative dementias [including AD, FTD, and dementia with Lewy bodies]."[3]

This consensus also states that "there is now agreement that cognitive impairments associated with cerebrovascular disease extend well beyond the traditional concept of multi-infarct dementia."[3] Another conclusion is that "memory impairment is not necessarily a prime symptom in vascular dementia." This 2003 consensus also proposed "use of the term *vascular cognitive impairment*…which is

TABLE 3–5.   Classification and causes of sporadic vascular cognitive impairment (O'Brien et al.[3])
Poststroke dementia
Vascular dementia
Multi-infarct dementia (cortical vascular dementia)
Subcortical ischemic vascular dementia
Strategic-infarct dementia
Hypoperfusion dementia
Hemorrhagic dementia
Dementia caused by specific arteriopathies
Mixed Alzheimer's disease and vascular dementia
Vascular mild cognitive impairment

characterized by a specific cognitive profile involving preserved memory with impairments in attention and executive functioning." The proposed classification of this vascular cognitive impairment entity is shown in Table 3–5.

Dementia in Pick's Disease

The ICD-10 defines dementia in Pick's disease as "a progressive dementia, commencing in middle age, characterized by early, slowly progressing changes of character and social deterioration, followed by impairment of the intellect, memory, and language functions, with apathy, euphoria and, occasionally, extrapyramidal phenomena" (F02.0).

DSM-IV-TR defines dementia attributable to Pick's disease as follows: "Pick's disease is characterized clinically by changes in personality early in the course, deterioration in social skills, emotional blunting, behavioral disinhibition, and prominent language abnormalities. Difficulties with memory, apraxia, and other features of dementia usually follow later in the course." DSM-IV-TR also notes that this condition is "one of the pathologically distinct etiologies among the heterogeneous group of dementing processes that are associated with frontotemporal brain atrophy." Despite this nascent recognition of FTD in DSM-IV-TR, the document continues as follows: "Dementia due to frontotemporal degeneration other than Pick's disease should be diagnosed as Dementia Due to Frontotemporal Degeneration, one of the dementias due to other general medical conditions."

A modern view of the above definitions would be that for both ICD-10 and DSM-IV-TR, the terminology and classification of this entity should be broadened in future diagnostic manuals to the term *frontotemporal dementias*. The Association for Frontotemporal Dementias (AFTD; http://www.ftd-picks.org) defines

---

TABLE 3–6.   Frontotemporal dementia: subtypes from the Association for
Frontotemporal Dementias (AFTD)

Pick's disease

FTDP-17 (frontotemporal dementia with parkinsonism linked to
chromosome 17)

Corticobasal degeneration

Progressive aphasia

Semantic dementia

Neurofibrillary tangle dementia

---

these entities as "neurodegenerative disorders primarily affect[ing] the frontal and
anterior regions of the brain. These areas control 'executive functions' involved in
reasoning and decision-making, planning, personality and social behavior, and
speech and language comprehension." Included in FTD are the conditions listed
in Table 3–6.

Another aspect of the critique of the DSM-IV-TR definition is that the general
dementia inclusion criterion of "memory impairment" excludes many FTD patients
until relatively late in the progression of their condition. The AFTD notes that
"memory loss…emerges later in these conditions." An FTD consensus from 1998 also
noted that "the most common clinical manifestation of FTLD [frontotemporal lobar
dementia] is with relative preservation of memory function (FTD)."[4]

Dementia in Parkinson's Disease and Lewy Body Dementia

ICD-10 has a category "dementia in Parkinson's disease" (F02.3). It is noted that
"no particular distinguishing clinical features have yet been demonstrated" for this
entity. There is no mention of Lewy body disease (LBD) here.

DSM-IV-TR describes an entity "dementia due to Parkinson's disease" (294.1x).
It is noted that "the dementia…is characterized by cognitive and motoric slowing,
executive dysfunction, and impairment in memory retrieval." DSM-IV-TR further notes that "dementia due to Lewy Body Disease in the absence of evidence of
Parkinson's…should be diagnosed as due to Lewy Body Disease, one of the dementias due to other general medical conditions."

A current critique would include the statement that LBD would appear to be
misclassified as a general medical condition. However, the validity of LBD remains
in doubt. Some have noted that the effects of parkinsonian treatment for this condition with dopaminergic agonists, such as levodopa and carbidopa, may produce
the visual hallucinations that have been said to be characteristic of Lewy body dis-

ease. These "therapeutic" agents may also be responsible for the sleep disruption of LBD. The parkinsonian features characteristic of LBD may account for the neuroleptic sensitivity.[39]

With regard to the more general entity of "dementia due to Parkinson's disease," current studies appear to indicate that the terminology "dementia associated with Parkinson's disease" might be a more appropriate nomenclature. For example, a recent study found close relationships between standard global and functional assessments of AD course and the evolution of loss of cognition and dementia in patients with Parkinson's disease.[40] The implication of these findings and related findings for many investigators is that this entity is, in reality, the concurrence, perhaps by chance in aged subjects, of AD with Parkinson's disease. If this is correct, then the term "dementia due to Parkinson's disease" from DSM-IV-TR would not be appropriate.

Other Dementias

Both DSM-IV-TR and ICD-10 list several other conditions that produce dementia under major etiopathogenic headings. A complete review of these other categories is well beyond the scope of this brief commentary. However, some succinct comments will be noted.

DSM-IV-TR notes the following additional categories: dementia due to other general medical conditions; dementia due to HIV disease; dementia due to head trauma; dementia due to Huntington's disease; substance-induced persisting dementia; dementia due to multiple etiologies; and dementia not otherwise specified. With minor caveats with respect to terminology, the retention of these other categories is endorsed. The minor caveats with respect to nomenclature include the following:

1. The word "general" in the category "other general medical conditions" appears to be superfluous, at best, and possibly misleading. The misleading element is related to the listing of primary brain disorders, such as Lewy body dementia, and frontotemporal dementia, among others, in this category (p. 167).
2. The terminology "dementia due to prion disease" should probably replace the category "dementia due to Creutzfeldt-Jakob disease."

ICD-10 also lists many of the same other dementia categories as DSM-IV-TR. Consequently, the same endorsements and caveats apply. The ICD-10 category of "dementia in other specified diseases classified elsewhere" can be endorsed. The ICD-10 does not have a category "dementia due to multiple etiologies," and this is a deficiency.

Future Directions

The current diagnostic descriptions are invaluable in that they provide a fertile substrate for a more current diagnostic nomenclature. However, in the dementia field, the diagnostic manuals have sometimes lagged by many years and even decades behind current scientific discoveries. An example of this temporal lag is the presenile/senile dementia dichotomy reviewed in some detail in this book. Similarly, there have been numerous studies of the symptomatic manifestations of AD, the major form of dementia pathology, as it evolves through all of the stages. Future classifications should use current knowledge of the symptomatology of AD. As noted, current consensus are unanimous in the conclusion that AD can be recognized for its characteristic symptomatology. These consensus have been arrived at as a result of extensive research. A few examples of such research are worthy of citation.

Staging procedures for dementia in general—notably the Clinical Dementia Rating (CDR)[41] and, for AD somewhat more specifically, the Global Deterioration Scale[42]—were developed in the early part of the 1980s and subsequently have been widely used and validated. The CDR staging was elaborated on by Morris[43] in 1993. The GDS was elaborated into a staging system, with additional elements that have been demonstrated to be optimally concordant with the GDS over the course of AD, including the Brief Cognitive Rating Scale (BCRS)[44] and the Functional Assessment Staging (FAST) procedure.[45] Each element of the GDS/BCRS/FAST staging system has demonstrated reliability, construct validity, and criterion validity in terms of relationship to AD neuropathology and/or sensitivity to pharmacotherapeutic intervention.

These scales have also been widely used. For example, the Alzheimer's Association uses and disseminates the GDS staging procedure to assist family members and professionals around the world in understanding the nature and course of AD.[46] The FAST staging procedure is mandated by the U.S. government for certain purposes.[47] All of the elements of the GDS/BCRS/FAST staging system have been used in the worldwide approvals of two of the four currently marketed Alzheimer's medications (memantine and rivastigmine). These descriptions, together with other worldwide research on the nature of the clinical presentation of AD, can be used to inform a more specific description of AD, as a diagnosis of inclusion, for DSM-V. Given the dramatically different nature of AD as it evolves, it is recommended that this description of AD incorporate available knowledge of the stages of the disease entity.

This summary of diagnostic criteria in dementia is being written several years before the advent of DSM-V. Consequently, it is appropriate to recommend research that might be accomplished over the next few years that could inform the DSM-V description of the dementia entities. Two such research procedures are recommended.

One procedure is to exploit recent developments in the in vivo and genetic-diagnosis of the dementias—using, for example, cerebrospinal fluid tau and β-amyloid (Aβ) markers—to examine the utility of clinical descriptions in the differentiation of the dementias. For example, patients with FTDs present with a different functional and behavioral profile of onset, in comparison with the magnitude of cognitive deficit, than do patients with AD. If we use existing measures that have been validated in the stage-specific description of the course of AD, these differences in clinical presentation for the subtypes of FTD can be elaborated on and confirmed.

A second research endeavor that can be commended also takes advantage of the relatively large body of clinical/behavioral research that has been conducted on AD over the past few decades. This research would be used to validate any proposed clinical descriptions for the non-AD dementia entities against actual informant and/or blinded clinician assessments of symptomatology.

In a paradigmatic study using these procedures, John Overall, the developer of a very widely used schizophrenia scale, and his colleagues[48] took 30 clinical elements of the description of the AD course from the GDS[42] and had relatives and caregivers of elderly patients in a clinic assess the presence or absence of each of the symptoms. Using statistical techniques of principal components analysis, these researchers recreated a scale based on the informant responses. They found that the clinical symptoms were observed to cluster into naturally occurring stages or phases. The occurrence of the stages or phases very closely mirrored the GDS staging descriptions. This approach to clinical validation by Overall and associates, which has been successful for AD, might be commended in the validation of emerging descriptions of putative symptomatology for the non-Alzheimer's dementias.

Another future direction is for the proposed dementia criteria to incorporate the emerging knowledge regarding the predementia clinical syndromes. Current diagnostic nosologies have recognized the existence of these predementia conditions.

For example, DSM-IV-TR refers to one of these conditions in "Appendix B: Criteria Sets and Axes Provided for Further Study." In this section, "mild neurocognitive disorder" is described in more than two pages (pp. 762–764). The DSM-IV-TR "research criteria for mild neurocognitive disorder" are generally consistent with prior descriptions of mild cognitive impairment (also referred to as *mild cognitive decline*) in the GDS staging (GDS stage 3).[42,49] Furthermore, in terms of inclusion and exclusion criteria, the DSM-IV-TR "research criteria for mild neurocognitive disorder" are quite similar to those suggested by Petersen and associates contemporaneously[50] and subsequently.[51] Aspects of the DSM-IV-TR "mild neurocognitive disorder description" which would likely be included in a present-day or future mild cognitive impairment nomenclature include 1) "memory impairment"; 2) "disturbance in executive functioning"; and 3) "impairment in social, occupational, or other important areas of functioning [which] represent a decline from a previous level of functioning."[1] The rationale for the inclusion of a mild cognitive impairment category in future nomenclatures has recently been reviewed.[52]

Depending on the setting, mild cognitive impairment may be viewed as a pre-dementia entity, generally a harbinger of Alzheimer's disease, or as a more diverse condition. In specialized memory clinic settings, a rate of progression of mild cognitive impairment subjects to Alzheimer's disease of 17% per year has been observed using the GDS stage 3 definition.[53] A virtually identical rate of progression (16%) has been noted using the Petersen amnestic mild cognitive impairment definition.[54] However, in more diverse clinical settings, "education, vascular risk factors, psychiatric status,...use of anticholinergic drugs," and many other conditions can influence the occurrence and course of mild cognitive impairment.[55]

DSM-IV-TR also has another category termed "age-related cognitive decline" (780.9) categorized as one of the "Other conditions that may be a focus of clinical attention." This condition requires "an objectively identified decline in cognitive functioning consequent to the aging process that is within normal limits given the person's age." Also, "individuals with this condition may report problems remembering names or appointments…"

The subjective deficits represented by this "age-related cognitive decline" condition have been described as stage 2 on the Global Deterioration Scale.[42] The Clinical Dementia Rating is silent as to the occurrence of these subjective complaints in older persons.[41] Nevertheless, these commonly occurring subjective impairments in normal older persons are increasingly being recognized as an important clinical entity, associated with an increased risk for dementia[56] and also for mild cognitive impairment.[57,58] Although the DSM-IV-TR-proposed criterion of an "objectively identified decline in cognitive functioning…that is within normal limits" remains an impractical standard (i.e., operational criteria for this standard do not exist at the present time), objective deficits in persons with these "normal" age-related cognitive complaints, in comparison with older persons without these complaints, have been demonstrated in terms of increased hippocampal atrophy,[59] increased electroencephalographic slow wave activity,[60] and increased urinary cortisol levels.[61] Terminologies that are currently being used for this seemingly prodromal stage of normal aging include "subjective cognitive impairment"[57] and subjective memory complaints.[61]

Future nomenclatures must also address the occurrence and nature of behavioral and psychological symptoms of dementia (BPSD). Current nomenclatures acknowledge these symptoms in the dementias. The ICD-10 notes that the dementias (F00–F03) "are commonly accompanied, and occasionally preceded, by deterioration in emotional control, social behavior, or motivation." However, with the exception of the category "dementia in Pick's disease," (F02.0), these emotional disturbances are not further addressed in the ICD-10.

The DSM-IV-TR notes behavioral disturbances and symptoms, both in the general context of the description of dementia and in the categorization of dementia types. In describing, "associated descriptive features" of dementia, the DSM-IV-

TR notes that "the multiple cognitive impairments of dementia are often associated with anxiety, mood and sleep disturbances. Delusions are common, especially those involving themes of persecution (e.g., that misplaced possessions have been stolen). Hallucinations can occur in all sensory modalities, but visual hallucinations are most common."[1(p.150)] This brief description is compatible with research findings (e.g., Reisberg et al. 1989[62]), with the caveat that the phrase "themes of persecution" is much too strong a descriptor for the nature of the symptoms manifested by patients. It is important that diagnostic manuals reflect genuine symptomatology and not take poetic license in the description of observed clinical phenomenon.

DSM-IV-TR also notes the presence or absence of behavioral disturbance in the coding of specific types of dementia. For example, for "dementia of the Alzheimer's type" subtypes "without behavioral disturbance," and "with behavioral disturbance" are coded. Also, other prominent clinical features can be indicated by coding on Axis I "for example, to indicate the presence of delusions,…depressed mood, and…persistent aggressive behavior."[1(p.155)] Vascular dementia and "dementia due to other general medical conditions" also have codes for the presence of behavioral disturbance.

Much research has been conducted on behavioral and psychological symptoms of dementia. For example, this work has been collected in two volumes from consensus conferences conducted by the International Psychogeriatric Association (IPA) in 1996[63] and in 1999.[64] The challenge for future nomenclatures is to express this detailed information in useful and meaningful ways for clinicians (see Chapter 6, "Diagnostic Categories and Criteria for Neuropsychiatric Syndromes in Dementia," this volume).[65]

Finally, there has been much discussion about the possibility of introducing a dimensional, rather than a categorical, classification for mental disorders. How well would this work for the dementias?

The answer appears to be "seemingly very well." For example, a functional severity dimension could be applied. One such functional severity dimensional measure that was briefly mentioned earlier in this chapter that is easy to administer, has been widely used worldwide, and has been extensively validated is the FAST procedure.[45] The FAST can be scored both for severity and for non-ordinal aspects, providing diagnostic information and cross diagnosis comparisons (e.g., in frontotemporal dementia and Alzheimer's disease). The severity comparisons would be very meaningful, for example, in terms of corresponding care needs.

Another possibility that has been discussed is a single category of dementia with differentiation of its types by a set of dimensions. This might also be feasible and possibly useful, with a few key dimensions such as magnitude of cognitive decline, magnitude of functional capacity, and magnitude of behavioral disturbances. The utility of this multidimensional approach might profitably be investigated in the next few years, or, alternatively, current knowledge and instruments could be judiciously applied.

Conclusion

Current diagnostic manuals are invaluable in presenting accumulated wisdom regarding dementia diagnosis. This area of scientific and clinical knowledge has been evolving very rapidly in recent years, concomitantly with the growth of the more general discipline of neuroscience. More recent, presently well-established information regarding Alzheimer's disease and other dementia entities should be incorporated in future nomenclature manuals, in particular DSM-V and ICD-11, now in the planning stages. In addition, research that might better inform such future descriptions could be conducted within the next few years. Modern science, research, and medical advances are clearly the product of an international enterprise. Hence, it will be increasingly important to involve the international organizations concerned with psychogeriatric and related disciplines in the further development of the proposal for both DSM and the ICD.

References

1. American Psychiatric Association: Diagnostic and Statistical Manual of Mental Disorders, 4th Edition, Text Revision. Washington, DC, American Psychiatric Association, 2000, pp 135–180.
2. World Health Organization: International Classification of Diseases, 10th Revision. Geneva, World Health Organization, 1992.
3. O'Brien JT, Erkinjuntti T, Reisberg B, et al: Vascular cognitive impairment. Lancet Neurol 2:98, 2003.
4. Neary D, Snowden JS, Gustafson L, et al: Frontotemporal lobar degeneration: a consensus on clinical diagnostic criteria. Neurology 51:1546–1554, 1998.
5. Gove PB (corporate author), Merriam-Webster (ed): Webster's Third New International Dictionary, Unabridged. Springfield, MA, Merriam-Webster, 1993.
6. Anderson DM (chief lexicographer): Dorland's Illustrated Medical Dictionary, 30th Edition. Philadelphia, PA, WB Saunders (Elsevier), 2003.
7. Reisberg B, Saeed MU: Alzheimer's disease, in Comprehensive Textbook of Geriatric Psychiatry, 3rd Edition. Edited by Sadovoy J, Jarvik LF, Grossberg GT, et al. New York, WW Norton, 2004, pp 449–509.
8. Hachinski VC, Lassen NA, Marshall J: Multi-infarct dementia, a cause of mental deterioration in the elderly. Lancet 2:207–210, 1974.
9. Roth M, Tomlinson BE, Blessed G: Correlation between scores for dementia and counts of "senile plaques" in cerebral gray matter of elderly subjects. Nature 209:109–110, 1966.
10. Blessed G, Tomlinson BE, Roth M: The association between quantitative measures of dementia and the senile change in the cerebral gray matter of elderly subjects. Br J Psychiatry 114:797–811, 1968.
11. Tomlinson BE, Blessed G, Roth M: Observations on the brains of non-demented old people. Neurol Sci 7:331–356, 1968.
12. Tomlinson BE, Blessed G, Roth M: Observations on the brains of demented old people. Neurol Sci 11:205–242, 1970.

13. Blocq P, Marinesco G: Sur lés lesions et la pathogénie de l'épilepsie dite essentielle. La Semaine médicale 12:445–446, 1892.

14. Redlich E: Über miliare Sklerose der Hirnrinde bei seniler Atrophie. Jahrbücher für Psychiatrie und Neurologie 17:208–216, 1898.

15. Alzheimer A: Über eine eigenartige Erkrankung der Hirnrinde. Allgemeine Zeitschrift für Psychiatrie und psychisch-gerichtlich e Medezin 64:146–148, 1907.

16. Grunthal E: Clinical and anatomical investigations on senile dementia. Zeitschrift für die gesampte Neurologie und Psychiatrie 111:763, 1927.

17. Gellerstedt N: Our knowledge of cerebral changes in normal involution of old age. Upsala-Lak/Foren Forh 38:193, 1933.

18. Margolis G: Senile cerebral disease: a critical survey of traditional concepts based upon observations with newer techniques. Lab Invest 8:335–370, 1959.

19. Hirano A, Zimmerman HM: Alzheimer's neurofibrillary changes: a topographic study. Arch Neurol 7:227–242, 1962.

20. Corsellis JAN, Evans PH: The relation of stenosis of the extracranial cerebral arteries to mental disorders and cerebral degeneration in old age. Proceedings of the Fifth International Congress of Neuropathology, 1965, p 546.

21. Corsellis JAN: Mental Illness and the Ageing Brain (Monogr No 9). London, Maudsley, 1962.

22. Dermaut B, Kumar-Singh S, Rademakers R, et al: Tau is central in the genetic Alzheimer-frontotemporal dementia spectrum. Trends Genet 21:664–672, 2005.

23. McKhann G, Drachman D, Folstein M, et al: Clinical diagnosis of Alzheimer's disease: report of the NINCDS-ADRDA Work Group under the auspices of Department of Health and Human Services Task Force on Alzheimer's Disease. Neurology 34:939–944, 1984.

24. Kahn RL, Goldfarb AI, Pollack M, et al: Brief objective measures for the determination of mental status in the aged. Am J Psychiatry 117:326–328, 1960.

25. Folstein MF, Folstein SE, McHugh PR: "Mini-Mental State": a practical method for grading the cognitive state of patients for the clinician. J Psychiatr Res 12:189–198, 1975.

26. Blessed G, Tomlinson BE, Roth M: The association between quantitative measures of dementia and the senile change in the cerebral gray matter of elderly subjects. Br J Psychiatry 114:797–811, 1968.

27. Shader RL, Harmatz JS, Salzman C: A new scale for assessment in geriatric populations: Sandoz Clinical Assessment—Geriatric (SCAG). J Am Geriatr Soc 22:107–113, 1974.

28. Reisberg B, Burns A, Brodaty H, et al: Diagnosis of Alzheimer's disease: report of an International Psychogeriatric Association Special Meeting Work Group under the cosponsorship of Alzheimer's Disease International, the European Federation of Neurological Societies, the World Health Organization, and the World Psychiatric Association. Int Psychogeriatr 9 (suppl 1):11–38, 1997.

29. Small GW, Rabins PV, Barry PP, et al: Diagnosis and treatment of Alzheimer disease and related disorders: consensus statement of the American Association for Geriatric Psychiatry, the Alzheimer's Association, and the American Geriatrics Society. JAMA 278:1363–1371, 1997.

30. Mohs R, Kim G, Johns C, et al: Assessing changes in Alzheimer's disease: memory and language, in Handbook for Clinical Memory Assessment of Older Adults. Edited by Poon LW. Washington, DC, American Psychological Association, 1986, pp 149–155.

31. Wilson R, Kaszniak A: Longitudinal changes: progressive idiopathic dementia, in Handbook for Clinical Memory Assessment of Older Adults. Edited by Poon LW. Washington, DC, American Psychological Association, 1986, pp 285–293.

32. Auer SR, Sclan SG, Yaffee RA, et al: The neglected half of Alzheimer disease: cognitive and functional concomitants of severe dementia. J Am Geriatr Soc 42:1266–1272, 1994.

33. Reisberg B, Ferris SH, Torossian C, et al: Pharmacologic treatment of Alzheimer's disease: a methodologic critique based upon current knowledge of symptomatology and relevance for drug trials. Int Psychogeriatr 4 (suppl 1):9–42, 1992.

34. Cole MG, Dastoor DP, Koszycki D: The Hierarchic Dementia Scale. J Clin Exp Gerontol 5:219–234, 1983.

35. Wechsler DA: The Measurement and Appraisal of Adult Intelligence. Baltimore, MD, Williams & Wilkins, 1958.

36. Reisberg B, Ferris SH, de Leon MJ, et al: Stage-specific behavioral, cognitive, and in vivo changes in community residing subjects with age-associated memory impairment and primary degenerative dementia of the Alzheimer type. Drug Dev Res 15:101–114, 1988.

37. Franssen EH, Reisberg B, Kluger A, et al: Cognition independent neurologic symptoms in normal aging and probable Alzheimer's disease. Arch Neurol 48:148–154, 1991.

38. Franssen EH, Kluger A, Torossian CL, et al: The neurologic syndrome of severe Alzheimer's disease: relationship to functional decline. Arch Neurol 50:1029–1039, 1993.

39. Serby M, Samuels S: Diagnostic criteria for dementia with Lewy bodies reconsidered. Am J Geriatr Psychiatry 9:212–216, 2001.

40. Sabbagh MN, Silverberg N, Bircea S, et al: Is the functional decline of Parkinson's disease similar to the functional decline of Alzheimer's disease? Parkinsonism Relat Disord 11:311–315, 2005.

41. Hughes CP, Berg L, Danziger WL, et al: A new clinical scale for the staging of dementia. Br J Psychiatry 140:566–572, 1982.

42. Reisberg B, Ferris SH, de Leon MJ, et al: The Global Deterioration Scale for assessment of primary degenerative dementia. Am J Psychiatry 139:1136–1139, 1982.

43. Morris JC: The Clinical Dementia Rating (CDR): current version and scoring rules. Neurology 43:2412–2414, 1993.

44. Reisberg B, Ferris SH: The Brief Cognitive Rating Scale (BCRS). Psychopharmacol Bull 24:629–636, 1988.

45. Sclan SG, Reisberg B: Functional Assessment Staging (FAST) in Alzheimer's disease: reliability, validity and ordinality. Int Psychogeriatr 4 (suppl 1):55–69, 1992.

46. Alzheimer's Association. Available at: http://alz.org/AboutAD/stages.asp. Accessed February 10, 2006.

47. Health Care Financing Administration (HCFA): Hospice-Determining Terminal Status in Non-Cancer Diagnoses—Dementia, Policy Number (YPF #163) (Y Med #20). The Medicare News Brief (A Publication for All Medicare Part B Providers). September 1998; MNB–98-7. For current reference, see Centers for Medicare and Medicaid Services (CMS), Medicare Coverage Database, LCD for Hospice Alzheimer's Disease and Related Disorders (L16343). Available at: www.cms.gov.

48. Overall JE, Scott J, Rhoades HM: Empirical scaling of the stages of cognitive decline in senile dementia. J Geriatr Psychiatry Neurol 3:212–220, 1990.

49. Flicker C, Ferris SH, Reisberg B: Mild cognitive impairment in the elderly: predictors of dementia. Neurology 41:1006–1009, 1991.

50. Petersen RC, Smith GE, Waring SC, et al: Mild cognitive impairment clinical characterization and outcome. Arch Neurol 56:303–308, 1999.

51. Petersen RC: Mild cognitive impairment as a diagnostic entity. J Intern Med 256:183–194, 2004.

52. Petersen RC, O'Brien J: Mild cognitive impairment should be considered for DSM-V. J Geriatr Psychiatry Neurol 19:147–154, 2006.

53. Kluger A, Ferris SH, Golomb J, et al: Neuropsychological prediction of decline to dementia in nondemented elderly. J Geriatr Psychiatry Neurol 12:168–179, 1999.

54. Petersen RC, Thomas RG, Grundman M, et al: Vitamin E and donepezil for the treatment of mild cognitive impairment. N Engl J Med 352:2379–2388, 2005.

55. Gauthier S, Reisberg B, Zaudig M, et al: Mild cognitive impairment. Lancet 367:1262–1270, 2006.

56. Jorm AF, Christensen H, Korten AE, et al: Memory complaints as a precursor of memory impairment in older people: a longitudinal analysis over 7–8 years. Psychol Med 31:441–449, 2001.

57. Reisberg B, Ferris SH, de Leon MJ, et al: Subjective cognitive impairment: the premild cognitive impairment stage of brain degeneration: longitudinal outcome after a mean of 7 years follow-up. Neuropsychopharmacology 30 (suppl 1), S81, 2005.

58. Prichep LS, John ER, Ferris SH, et al: Prediction of longitudinal cognitive decline in normal elderly using electrophysiological imaging. Neurobiol Aging 27:471–481, 2006.

59. Saykin AJ, Wishart HA, Rabin LA, et al: Older adults with cognitive complaints show brain atrophy similar to that of amnestic MCI. Neurology 67:834–842, 2006.

60. Prichep LS, John ER, Ferris SH, et al: Quantitative EEG correlates of cognitive deterioration in the elderly. Neurobiol Aging 15:85–90, 1994.

61. Wolf OT, Dziobek I, McHugh P, et al: Subjective memory complaints in aging are associated with elevated cortisol levels. Neurobiol Aging 26:1357–1363, 2005.

62. Reisberg B, Franssen E, Sclan SG, et al: Stage specific incidence of potentially remediable behavioral symptoms in aging and Alzheimer's disease: a study of 120 patients using the BEHAVE-AD. Bulletin of Clinical Neurosciences 54:95–112, 1989.

63. Finkel SI (ed): Behavioral and psychological signs and symptoms of dementia: implications for research and treatment. Int Psychogeriatr 8 (suppl 3):215–552, 1996.

64. Finkel SI, Burns A (eds): Behavioral and psychological symptoms of dementia (BPSD): a clinical and research update. Int Psychogeriatr 12 (suppl 1):9–424, 2000.

65. Finkel SI, Costa e Silva J, Cohen G, et al: Behavioral and psychological signs and symptoms of dementia: a consensus statement on current knowledge and implications for research and treatment. Int Psychogeriatr 8 (suppl 3):497–500, 1996.

Appendix
Summary of Recommendations of Changes for DSM-V

Overall rubric of the dementias
The organic/nonorganic dichotomy should be abandoned.[a]
The general term *cognitive disorders* should be considered for these conditions.[a]

Definition of dementia
The acquired nature of these conditions should be noted.[b]
The generalized nature of the occurrence and evolution of cognitive deficits, which, in progressive dementias, may present initially in diverse ways, depending in part on the nature of the dementia disorder, should be emphasized. Memory deficit should not be overemphasized. The prominence of early (diagnostic) deficits in aphasia, apraxia, and agnosia, as opposed to generalized cognition deficits, should not be overemphasized.[b]
The occurrence of progressive changes in functional capacities should be noted.[a]
The frequent occurrence of personality and behavior changes should also be noted.[b]

Alzheimer's disease
The dichotomy with age at onset of age 65 should be abandoned.[a]
The clinical features of Alzheimer's disease should be described.[a]
The emphasis that "dementia of Alzheimer's type" is a diagnosis of exclusion should be abandoned.[b]
The course of Alzheimer's disease should be described, incorporating current knowledge.[a]

Vascular dementia
The central concept of vascular dementia as being primarily related to multiple infarctions should probably be placed within a much broader concept of vascular disease–related cognitive impairment.[b]
The consensus vascular cognitive impairment nosologic entities should be given consideration.[a]

Pick's disease
The terminology should be broadened to the concept of frontotemporal dementia. This might include subcategories in addition to Pick's disease, such as frontotemporal dementia with parkinsonism linked to chromosome 17, corticobasal degeneration, and progressive aphasia.[a]

Dementia due to Parkinson's disease
The above terminology from DSM-IV-TR should be reconsidered.
A more accurate terminology might be "dementia associated with Parkinson's disease" or the term used by the ICD-10: "dementia in Parkinson's disease."[b]

Dementia due to other general medical conditions

The word "general" should be omitted from the above terminology.[b]

Mild neurocognitive disorder

Currently classified in Appendix B: Criteria Sets and Axes Provided for Further
    Study," this condition should be moved to a more formal diagnostic category.[b]

The terminology might be modified to the presently more widely used term
    "mild cognitive impairment."[a]

Age-related cognitive decline

Currently classified under "other conditions that may be a focus of clinical
    attention," this condition currently requires "an objectively identified decline in
    cognitive functioning...that is within normal limits given the person's age," an
    impossible standard in the current state of practice and knowledge.[b]

This condition should be reclassified and reconceptualized as "subjective
    cognitive impairment," or under an equivalent term, recognizing that the
    primary clinical manifestation is subjective impairment.[a]

Universal dementia comparators

A severity dimension, such as the magnitude of functional impairment, might be
    employed for cross-diagnostic severity comparisons.[a]

Alternatively, multiple severity dimensions such as (a) cognitive and functional,
    or (b) cognitive, functional, and behavioral dimensions, might be employed for
    cross-diagnostic severity comparisons.[a]

---

[a]Recommendation of change refers primarily to both DSM-IV-TR and ICD-10.
[b]Recommendation of change refers primarily to DSM-IV-TR.

4

MILD COGNITIVE IMPAIRMENT SHOULD BE CONSIDERED FOR DSM-V

Ronald C. Petersen, Ph.D., M.D.
John O'Brien, D.M., F.R.C.Psych.

Should mild cognitive impairment (MCI) be considered as a diagnostic entity in the *Diagnostic and Statistical Manual of Mental Disorders*, 5th Edition (DSM-V)? We would like to make a case for this possibility. With increasing diagnostic sophistication among clinicians and the need for identifying disease processes at the earliest point in time, MCI has become a useful construct. In fact, MCI is being used both in clinical practice and in research, and, consequently, it appears that clinicians/investigators are finding the entity useful. It then becomes important for those involved in the development of DSM-V to consider whether there is sufficient evidence to consider codifying MCI.

As consideration is given to the development of DSM-V, several important issues need to be addressed. Initially, who is the audience? If the answer to this question pertains to academic psychiatrists, then one set of criteria can be developed in-

Supported in part by the National Institute on Aging, Mayo Clinic Alzheimer's Disease Research Center (P50 AG16574), Mayo Clinic Alzheimer's Disease Patient Registry (U01 AG06786), Alzheimer's Disease Cooperative Study (U01 AG10483), and Robert H. and Clarice Smith and Abigail Van Buren Alzheimer's Disease Research Program.

This chapter is reprinted from Petersen RC, O'Brien J: "Mild Cognitive Impairment Should Be Considered for DSM-V." *Journal of Geriatric Psychiatry and Neurology* 19:147–154, 2006. Used with permission.

cluding state-of-the-art technology, neuroimaging, biomarkers, neuropsychological testing, and the like, which it is hoped will improve the sensitivity and specificity of diagnoses. However, if the criteria are meant to be used by virtually all clinicians, irrespective of the level of sophistication or access to technology, then different considerations apply. These criteria will need to be largely clinically based, with less reliance on technology.

Second, what is the gold standard for assessing the utility of the diagnoses defined by the criteria? Often in neuropsychiatric disorders, especially the dementias, many believe that the gold standard lies in neuropathology at the time of autopsy. However, although that is a commonly held belief, the criteria for pathological diagnoses for Alzheimer's disease (AD), vascular dementia, dementia with Lewy bodies, and frontotemporal dementia are in a state of flux; consequently, this issue is not simple. Moreover, because of the link between MCI and dementia, the natural assumption is that the gold standard for MCI, was with dementia, should be neuropathology. However, for the majority of disorders included in the DSM classification system, there is no known neuropathology. Therefore, to judge that MCI needs a neuropathological gold standard is to hold it to a much higher degree of rigor than is expected of most other psychiatric disorders, which, like MCI, are primarily validated because of their symptom profile, therapeutic response, and outcome. Consequently, the issue of a gold standard is not trivial. We will return to these issues after discussing issues concerning MCI.

What Is Mild Cognitive Impairment?

Mild cognitive impairment has come to represent a transitional state between the cognitive changes of aging and the earliest clinical features of dementia.[1,2] We emphasize the clinical features of dementia because some would contend that if a person has any of the neuropathological features of dementia such as AD, he or she should be designated as having AD at that point in time.[3] However, we would argue that unless we have extremely high specificities for our clinical criteria, presumptively labeling somebody with a suspected neuropathological diagnosis is premature at this point, and the enormous emotional and practical consequences of an erroneous diagnosis of early dementia are obvious.[4,5] Improved clinical criteria to enable the diagnosis to be made earlier will be important, but current clinical criteria are not sufficiently specific at this point to enable this.

Over the years, a variety of sets of terminology have been proposed to account for cognitive changes in aging.[6–9] Many of these terms, such as *benign senescent forgetfulness, age-associated memory impairment,* and *age-associated cognitive decline,* have been developed to describe the extremes of normal aging.[6,7] However, MCI is not an extension of normal aging; rather, it is meant to describe an early pathological condition that has sufficient specificity to lead to more severe dementing disorders.

Originally, the criteria for MCI focused on a memory disorder and the likelihood that this condition would progress to AD.[10] Most of the literature today still focuses on the amnestic form of MCI as a precursor to clinical AD.[11–13] However, others have noted that not all forms of MCI necessarily progress to AD, and the construct must be broadened.[14] In 2003, an international panel of experts was convened in Stockholm to consider the criteria and expand them to include other forms of cognitive impairment that may precede dementia.[15,16] These criteria have been published and have been adopted by the National Institute on Aging's Alzheimer's Disease Centers Program in its Uniform Data Set and by the National Institute on Aging–sponsored Alzheimer's Disease Neuroimaging Initiative.[17]

Mild Cognitive Impairment Vis à Vis Dementia (DSM-IV)

The evolution of the MCI criteria from being memory centered to being more inclusive of other forms of cognitive impairment may be a harbinger of what needs to be considered for DSM-V. That is, if dementia is meant to include all types of cognitive impairment involving multiple cognitive domains of sufficient severity to interfere with one's daily activities, then perhaps the memory requirement for dementia should also be reconsidered.[18] The criterion for memory impairment, although nearly always met in cases of AD, causes considerable problems and tautology when applied to vascular, frontotemporal, and Lewy body "dementias," when, despite multiple and severe cognitive deficits, memory impairment may not be prominent. One could envision a new definition of dementia referring to a state in which two or more cognitive domains are impaired to a sufficient degree to affect daily activities. Then once the diagnosis of dementia is made, more specific criteria can be applied to the subtypes of dementias such as AD, frontotemporal dementia, dementia with Lewy bodies, vascular cognitive impairment, and other dementias. In the same vein as the definition of dementia, MCI could then be a precursor of all forms of dementia that is more broadly defined, as was done following the Stockholm conference.[15]

This topic is not covered adequately in DSM-IV. That is, the only mild cognitive type of disorder in DSM-IV is "mild neurocognitive disorder," which refers to an impairment in two or more areas of cognition that is attributable to a medical disorder. This entity has not really been studied to any extent and is quite different from the MCI proposed here. There is a need in DSM-V to recognize earlier stages of the AD process, because patients are presenting at earlier time points and physicians are challenged with the appropriate recognition and treatment of this condition. Furthermore, with the increasing numbers of persons reaching the age of risk for dementia, this is going to become an increasingly important issue, and DSM-V should address it.

Why do we need a definition for dementia at all if we can make a more specific diagnosis concerning the subtypes of dementia such as AD? We think the answer to this question pertains to specificity. Although the diagnostic field has advanced greatly in recent years, we still cannot label with sufficient certainty every dementia encountered in practice with a specific subtype. That is, there is still a role for the diagnosis of dementia, perhaps "not otherwise specified." In the future, this term may be retired and replaced by a variety of specific subtypes of dementia, but at this point, we still need the general term because we cannot subclassify every type of cognitive impairment meeting dementia criteria into a specific subtype. In addition, subtype diagnosis of dementia depends on the point at which diagnosis is made, with evidence that diagnosis is more difficult in the very early and very late stages of dementia, when symptoms may be very similar, than in the middle stages, when the classic profile of different subtypes of dementia is more often seen. Therefore, we could propose a revision in DSM-V to include the term *dementia* whose definition begins with any type of cognitive impairment in two or more domains of sufficient severity to affect one's daily activities (Figure 4–1). Then, the next step in the diagnostic process would be to subclassify the dementia into a specific subtype, such as AD, if possible.

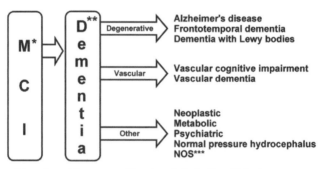

* Impairment in any cognitive domain but of insufficient severity to affect function

** Impairment in any 2 or more cognitive domains and sufficiently severe to affect function

*** Does not fit a known dementia syndrome

FIGURE 4–1.   Proposed scheme involving the progression of broadly defined types of mild cognitive impairment (MCI) to dementia and then the subclassification of particular types of dementia.

Source.   Reprinted from Petersen[46] with permission.

If dementia were to be expanded to include these considerations (e.g., lack of requirement of a memory deficit), then MCI could be a precursor stage. MCI in its broadest interpretation might include a cognitive complaint of any type and an impairment in a single cognitive domain but of insufficient severity to compromise daily function (Figure 4–1). This, of course, is a clinical judgment, but clinicians make these decisions on a regular basis with variable degrees of technological assistance and are quite accurate. The American Academy of Neurology, following an evidence-based medicine review of the literature, concluded that clinicians are actually quite accurate in making the diagnosis of dementia when they follow the current criteria proposed in DSM-IV.[19] Similarly, clinicians are quite accurate at making the clinical diagnosis of AD as well, and consequently, this same type of accuracy, with appropriate education, can be accomplished with MCI criteria.

Mild Cognitive Impairment Subtypes

At the Stockholm conference on MCI, the original MCI construct, which focused largely on memory, was expanded to include other types of cognitive impairments, because it was appreciated that not all forms of MCI go on to AD.[15] The scheme shown in Figure 4–2 was proposed to allow for any type of cognitive concern, with the subsequent subclassification of patients according to the memory domain into amnestic or nonamnestic subtypes and ultimately into single or multiple domain classifications of the amnestic and nonamnestic subtypes. This diagnostic scheme has been adopted by the National Institute on Aging's Alzheimer's Disease Centers Program through its Uniform Data Set and also by the Alzheimer's Disease Neuroimaging Initiative. The amnestic MCI (aMCI) arm of the diagram has been investigated to a much greater extent than has the nonamnestic MCI (naMCI) arm, and the latter may be more heuristic at this point.

Outcome

One of the primary means of establishing credibility for a clinical entity involves its ability to predict outcomes. In the case of MCI, the literature has been variable, but some order can be brought to these studies. If one classifies these studies on the basis of clinical populations, you will find clinic-based and population-based studies. In general, the clinic-based studies are more uniform and have led to the often quoted figures for progression of aMCI of 10%–15% per year.[10,11,13] This likely represents data from a subset of all MCI patients, but an important subset because these are the patients considered when more accurate diagnostic criteria are being generated. Again, this is quite similar to the manner in which DSM diagnoses should be made. If one were developing criteria for autism, you would not do a population-based study to investigate the issues; rather, you would find the purest cases in the clinic on which to develop your criteria.

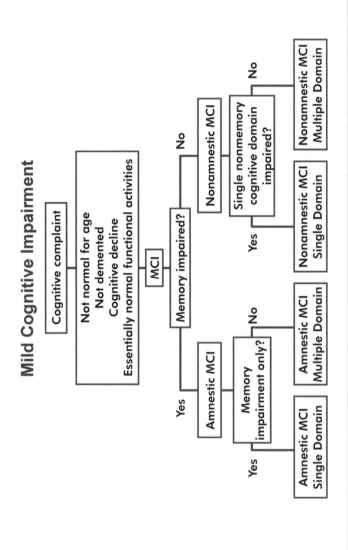

FIGURE 4–2.   Current diagnostic scheme for the diagnosis of mild cognitive impairment (MCI) and its subtypes.

Source.   Petersen.[16]

Criteria and outcomes for the nonamnestic types of MCI are less well studied and data are forthcoming.[20] Consequently, it is difficult to make a strong case for the inclusion of naMCI subtypes as DSM disorders.

The other major classes of outcome data are gathered by means of population-based studies, which can be subdivided into those that were done retrospectively (i.e., retrofitting MCI criteria to existing data sets) and prospective studies in which the MCI criteria were specified a priori. Several studies in the first category reported inconsistent data with variable outcomes of MCI patients over time.[21,22] Some of these noted reversion to normal rates in the range of 25%–40%.[22,23] However, when these studies are examined more closely, it is apparent that the entire definition of MCI may have depended on performance on a single neuropsychological test of memory.[22] That is, when inclusion in the study was based on performance on a single measure, one can envision inherent instability in the outcome. In the PAQUID study from France, MCI was based on a particular cutoff score on the Benton Visual Retention Test alone, and, consequently, when a patient scored just below the cutoff score on one occasion and just above the cutoff score on another occasion, that person would be described as reverting from MCI to normal.[22] This determination was made independently of the assessment of potential etiologies of the clinical syndrome. Factors such as psychiatric conditions, medication use, fatigue, and medical comorbidities were all lumped together in following these patients longitudinally as determined by the study design. As the authors have stated, the fluctuation in performance could be influenced by numerous factors, and these fluctuations do not necessarily have any implication for the underlying construct of MCI as a clinical entity; rather, they reflect neuropsychological variability across time. Consequently, many of the retrospectively designed population-based studies are informative, but the results need to be interpreted with caution.

In addition, many of these epidemiological studies, because of their designs, were unable to corroborate a subjective cognitive concern by an informant and were unable to document any type of decline in cognition, which put them at a disadvantage for fulfilling MCI criteria. Consequently, although many of these epidemiological studies have produced very useful information, they have not been able to address certain issues because these factors were not considered in the original design. Again, these are not flaws in the studies; rather, the studies were designed to address other questions, and the MCI issues were raised after the fact.

Prospectively designed epidemiological studies are likely to be more beneficial in shedding light on the time course of MCI, because the criteria are defined and the diagnoses are made a priori according to preestablished criteria. Several of these studies are beginning to emerge and are providing meaningful data, clearly showing that a diagnosis of MCI has important predictive validity.[11,12,24] Although not population-based, the Religious Order Study has produced important data on a prospectively designed cohort of patients with MCI.[13,25] These studies have shown that the amnestic form of MCI does progress to AD at an accelerated rate and that

MCI is associated with an increased risk of death.[11–13,26] A recent study from the Mayo Clinic has also shown that aMCI patients had a decreased survival and that between the aMCI subtypes, multiple domain aMCI had a poorer prognosis than single domain aMCI.[27]

Other prospective studies such as the Cache County Study, Mayo Clinic Study of Aging, University of Pittsburgh Monongahela Youghiogheny Healthy Aging Study, and Cardiovascular Health Study are under way and are likely to provide important data on the outcome of MCI.[11,28]

Kendell's Criteria

Some would argue that a disorder cannot be classified as such unless it meets a set of criteria such as Kendell's criteria.[29] Although this argument is intuitively reasonable, these criteria are somewhat arbitrary and the actual utility of these criteria is unknown. Most disorders classified in DSM-IV would likely not meet all these criteria, although we argue that MCI meets these criteria at least as well as, if not better than, many other disorders currently in DSM. The criteria are as follows:

1. *Clarity about the identification and description.*   Clear criteria for MCI have been established, are internationally used, and have been adopted by the National Institute on Aging's Alzheimer's Disease Centers Program for use in its Uniform Data Set and by the National Institute on Aging–funded trials such as the Alzheimer's Disease Cooperative Study Mild Cognitive Impairment Treatment Trial and the Alzheimer's Disease Neuroimaging Initiative.[17]
2. *Demonstration of a boundary or point of rarity between related syndromes.*   MCI can in fact be distinguished from normal aging by means of a clinical examination including an interview and neuropsychological testing. Similarly, it can be distinguished from AD by establishing the presence or absence of a loss of ability to perform activities of daily living.[30,31]
3. *A distinct course.*   Amnestic MCI progresses to AD at a predictable rate of 10%–15% per year in many studies.[10,11]
4. *A distinct treatment response.*   One clinical trial suggested that a cholinesterase inhibitor may reduce the rate at which MCI progresses to AD; however, there are no accepted treatments at this point in time.[32,33] However, this possible effect does not distinguish MCI from AD, many other dementing illnesses, or other psychiatric conditions in DSM-IV. In addition, most of the acetylcholinesterase inhibitor trials in MCI have been negative except for the partially positive effect found in the Alzheimer's Disease Cooperative Study of donepezil and vitamin E, implying that perhaps different therapies are needed for aMCI than for AD because of the distinctiveness of the disorders.[33]

5. *A clear association with a fundamental abnormality.*   Patients with MCI demonstrate a number of abnormalities compared with similar-aged control participants, including hypoperfusion and hypometabolism on functional brain imaging studies (functional magnetic resonance imaging and positron emission tomography), hippocampal and medial temporal lobe changes on magnetic resonance imaging, and cerebrospinal fluid changes in tau and Aβ amyloid. Several studies concerning the neuropathological substrate of aMCI have been published recently, indicating that most likely the pathology is intermediate between the changes of normal aging and the very earliest features of AD.[3–5] Most disorders in DSM-IV do not have known neuropathology.

6. *A genetic pattern.*   Amnestic MCI has a similar genetic profile to that of AD, with *APOE* ε4 carrier status being a risk factor.[33–35]

Therefore, aMCI does meet most of Kendell's criteria and can be considered a valid disorder.

Where Are We?

STRENGTHS

The current diagnostic scheme for MCI (Figure 4–2) can be applied by most physicians in a uniform fashion. Several large clinical trials have been completed, and a reasonably uniform set of patients has been recruited.[32,33,36] As mentioned, the National Institute on Aging's Alzheimer's Disease Centers Program uses these criteria, as does the Alzheimer's Disease Neuroimaging Initiative for aMCI, and there is acceptance among the clinicians. The American Academy of Neurology performed an evidence-based medicine review of the literature and concluded that MCI is a useful clinical construct and that clinicians should identify these patients and monitor them for their increased risk of developing a subsequent dementia.[37]

Although the outcomes are somewhat variable, as described earlier, when certain constraints are placed on the studies (e.g., clinic-based or prospectively designed MCI epidemiology studies), the outcomes are much more uniform.[10] If aMCI criteria are applied in conjunction with assessment of the proposed etiology of the condition, there is good agreement on the likelihood of progression to AD.[16] In addition, there are certain features that tend to predict a more rapid progression from aMCI to AD, such as *APOE* ε4 carrier status and atrophic hippocampal formation volumes on magnetic resonance imaging.[35,38–41] We are hearing more about putative predictors such as biomarkers—for example, cerebrospinal fluid tau and Aβ, and possibly amyloid imaging.[42–44] These are studies for the future.

The diagnosis of MCI can be made by most clinicians in much the same fashion as making the diagnosis of dementia or AD. Thresholds need to be adjusted, but otherwise the same principles apply. Neuropsychological testing can be very helpful in making the clinical judgment, but it must be emphasized that this is not a neuropsychological diagnosis. That is, there are no "MCI tests" or cutoff scores that determine the diagnosis; it is a judgment call on the part of the clinician in the same fashion as one would make the diagnosis of dementia or AD.

WEAKNESSES

Until clinicians become more comfortable with making diagnostic calls at an earlier point in the disease spectrum, there will be hesitation on the part of some. This may gradually resolve with education and familiarity with making these diagnoses.

There are still challenges in operationalizing the criteria. Because cognitive testing does play an important role in the diagnostic decision-making process, variability in instruments, numbers of tests, cutoff scores, and normative data all become relevant issues. However, if one reverts to the point made earlier about the use of clinical judgment in fulfilling these criteria, these issues become less problematic.

Some of the MCI subtypes, such as naMCI, have not been validated. There are many more studies available on aMCI than on naMCI at this point, and, consequently, naMCI probably should remain a research entity worthy of further investigation.

Neuropathological data on MCI are increasing in the literature, but there is no consensus.[3–5] Some investigators believe that aMCI is already neuropathologically established AD, whereas others contend that the data imply an intermediate stage between the neuropathological findings of normal aging and very early AD.[3–5] Therefore, the issue of the gold standard with respect to these diagnoses once again becomes important to discuss, although as argued earlier in this chapter, the fact that MCI already has some evidence of neuropathological changes places it ahead of many psychiatric disorders that are already in DSM-IV.

Where Do We Go From Here?

Before we consider including MCI in DSM-V, additional research needs to be conducted. It is hoped that with more consistent use of the proposed set of criteria for MCI, outcome studies will be less variable. Many of the answers to key questions in the field are likely to be forthcoming in the ongoing longitudinal studies, as suggested in Table 4–1. Prospectively designed epidemiological studies should inform us on the prevalence of the condition and its subtypes, and longitudinal aging studies should give us important information on incidence as well. Preliminary data indicate that the prevalence of aMCI is probably twice that of AD for the appropriate ages, and the incidence rates are similar at approximately 1%–2% per year, but verification of these findings is essential.[10]

TABLE 4–1.   Proposed research on mild cognitive impairment (MCI)

Topic	Question	Studies needed
Clinical diagnoses	Refine aMCI criteria Develop naMCI construct	Prospective longitudinal studies
Outcome	aMCI: Improve specificity naMCI: Assess non-AD dementia outcomes	Prospective longitudinal studies
Predictors	Evaluate breadth of measures: clinical, genetic, imaging (structural, functional, amyloid), biomarkers to improve specificity of outcomes	Prospective longitudinal studies with imaging and biomarkers (e.g., ADNI)
Neuropathology	Determine the gold standard Redefine criteria	Consensus panels on neuropathological parameters Clinical trials in MCI
Therapeutics	Develop alternative therapies Use predictors above to enhance specificity	Clinical trials

Note.   ADNI=Alzheimer's Disease Neuroimaging Initiative; aMCI=amnestic MCI; naMCI=nonamnestic MCI.

These studies as well as clinic-based studies should inform us on the boundaries between normal aging and MCI, on the one hand, and between MCI and AD, on the other. This will take a sharpening of clinic acumen, but that is likely to evolve with increased experience in diagnosing clinical conditions at this stage in the disease process.

We need to expand our knowledge about predictors of progression. Will technology such as neuroimaging and biomarkers help us make the prediction? Do we know enough about the sensitivity and specificity of biomarkers to inform ourselves about the rates of progression? Longitudinal studies will help us address these issues.

We need more pathological data, but as indicated above, the interpretation of these data is not trivial. The variable thresholds in neuropathology may reflect the underlying predisposition of investigators with respect to their thresholds for calling the neuropathological diagnosis of AD. There is always a selection bias involving which patients come to autopsy and which do not. All of these issues must be addressed.

Original Questions

Returning to the original question, do we need two sets of criteria? It might be that a set of clinical criteria for MCI can be put forth along the lines of the criteria proposed in Stockholm and should be evaluated for their ultimate sensitivity and specificity. These would be applicable to all physicians to use regardless of access to various states of technology.

In addition, research criteria could be proposed that expand on the clinical criteria described above. That is, in addition to the clinical criteria, the added utility of neuroimaging, biomarkers, genotyping, and other measures can be tested to see if there is an improvement in the sensitivity and specificity of the outcomes. One would hypothesize that specificity, and perhaps sensitivity, may well be improved by the addition of these disease-specific tools. However, we may need to stop short of including these technological advances as part of the diagnostic criteria, because all clinicians may not have access to this degree of technology.

The question of a gold standard is difficult.[45] Although one can argue for the importance of neuropathological confirmation, this may not be the best solution. Ultimately, the best gold standard may be the clinical outcome of the entity. That is, if a condition can predict with reasonable certainty a clinical outcome, this may be the best set of criteria to assess its utility. It is hoped that this type of standard would then be modifiable with appropriate treatments. Although attempts to determine the underlying neuropathological substrate of a disorder are no doubt laudable, improving clinical function may be a more worthy measure of ultimate utility.

Conclusion

Mild cognitive impairment, at least amnestic MCI, should receive serious consideration for inclusion in DSM-V. Without any formal codification of criteria in any standard manual, the construct has been adopted by many clinicians and investigators as a useful construct. On the research side, hundreds of papers have been published with *mild cognitive impairment* in the title or abstract in the past 5 years, as is shown in Figure 4–3. The concept of MCI has influenced virtually all aspects of research on aging and dementia, including clinical aspects, neuropsychology, epidemiology, neuroimaging, neuropathology, mechanisms of disease, and clinical trials. The influence of a prodromal state of AD on these areas of investigation has been very informative.

On the clinical side, MCI is being used in practice. Clinicians find the construct useful and have no difficulty recognizing patients in this intermediate state. The challenge is in establishing specific criteria that are meaningful and predictive. Ultimately, if treatments become available, establishment of such criteria will be-

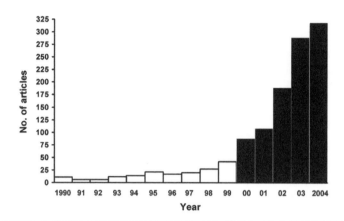

FIGURE 4–3.   Number of publications with *mild cognitive impairment* in either the title or the abstract from 1990 through 2004.

come an even more pressing need. As mentioned above, the American Academy of Neurology has already recommended to its clinicians that MCI is an important construct.[37]

Therefore, it appears that DSM-V can provide the clinical and research community a valuable service by codifying the disorder. Research on specific features of the criteria, leading to a refinement, may be necessary over the next several years to improve the sensitivity and specificity of the outcome.

References

1. Petersen RC: Conceptual overview, in Mild Cognitive Impairment: Aging to Alzheimer's Disease. Edited by Petersen RC. New York, Oxford University Press, 2003, pp 1–14.
2. Petersen RC, Doody R, Kurz A, et al: Current concepts in mild cognitive impairment. Arch Neurol 58:1985–1992, 2001.
3. Markesbery WR, Schmitt FA, Kryscio RJ, et al: Neuropathologic substrate of mild cognitive impairment. Arch Neurol 63:38–46, 2006.
4. Petersen RC, Parisi JE, Dickson DW, et al: Neuropathology of amnestic mild cognitive impairment. Arch Neurol 63:665–672, 2006.
5. Jicha GA, Parisi JE, Dickson DW, et al: Neuropathological outcome of mild cognitive impairment following progression to clinical dementia. Arch Neurol 63:674–681, 2006.
6. Kral VA: Senescent forgetfulness: benign and malignant. Can Med Assoc J 86:257–260, 1962.
7. Crook T, Bartus RT, Ferris SH, et al: Age-associated memory impairment: proposed diagnostic criteria and measures of clinical change—report of a National Institute of Mental Health work group. Dev Neuropsychol 2:261–276, 1986.

8. LaRue A: Aging and Neuropsychological Assessment. New York, Plenum, 1992.

9. Levy R: Aging-associated cognitive decline. Int Psychogeriatr 6:63–68, 1994.

10. Petersen RC, Smith GE, Waring SC, et al: Mild cognitive impairment: clinical characterization and outcome. Arch Neurol 56:303–308, 1999.

11. Lopez OL, Jagust WJ, DeKosky ST, et al: Prevalence and classification of mild cognitive impairment in the Cardiovascular Health Study Cognition Study. Arch Neurol 60:1385–1389, 2003.

12. Ganguli M, Dodge HH, Shen C, et al: Mild cognitive impairment, amnestic type: an epidemiologic study. Neurology 63:115–121, 2004.

13. Bennett DA, Wilson RS, Schneider JA, et al: Natural history of mild cognitive impairment in older persons. Neurology 59:198–205, 2002.

14. Gauthier S, Reisberg B, Zaudig M, et al: Mild cognitive impairment. Lancet 367: 1262–1270, 2006.

15. Winblad B, Palmer K, Kivipelto M, et al: Mild cognitive impairment—beyond controversies, towards a consensus. J Intern Med 256:240–246, 2004.

16. Petersen RC: Mild cognitive impairment as a diagnostic entity. J Intern Med 256:183–194, 2004.

17. Mueller SG, Weiner MW, Thal LJ, et al: Ways towards an early diagnosis in Alzheimer's disease: the Alzheimer's Disease Neuroimaging Initiative (ADNI). Alzheimer's & Dementia 1:55–66, 2005.

18. American Psychiatric Association: Diagnostic and Statistical Manual of Mental Disorders, 4th Edition. Washington, DC, American Psychiatric Association, 1994.

19. Knopman DS, DeKosky ST, Cummings JL, et al: Practice parameter: diagnosis of dementia (an evidence-based review): report of the Quality Standards Subcommittee of the American Academy of Neurology. Neurology 56:1143–1153, 2001.

20. Boeve BF, Ferman TJ, Smith GE, et al: Mild cognitive impairment preceding dementia with Lewy bodies. Neurology 62 (suppl 5):A86, 2004.

21. Ritchie K, Artero S, Touchon J: Classification criteria for mild cognitive impairment: a population-based validation study. Neurology 56:37–42, 2001.

22. Larrieu S, Letenneur L, Orgogozo JM, et al: Incidence and outcome of mild cognitive impairment in a population-based prospective cohort. Neurology 59:1594–1599, 2002.

23. Unverzagt FW, Gao S, Baiyewu O, et al: Prevalence of cognitive impairment: data from the Indianapolis Study of Health and Aging. Neurology 57:1655–1662, 2001.

24. Lopez OL, Jagust WJ, Dulberg C, et al: Risk factors for mild cognitive impairment in the Cardiovascular Health Study Cognition Study. Arch Neurol 60:1394–1399, 2003.

25. Bennett DA, Schneider JA, Bienias JL, et al: Mild cognitive impairment is related to Alzheimer disease pathology and cerebral infarctions. Neurology 64:834–841, 2005.

26. Fisk JD, Merry HR, Rockwood K: Variations in case definition affect prevalence but not outcomes of mild cognitive impairment. Neurology 61:1179–1184, 2003.

27. Hunderfund AL, Roberts RO, Slusser TC, et al: Mortality in amnestic mild cognitive impairment: a prospective community study. Neurology 67:1764–1768, 2006.

28. Zandi PP, Anthony JC, Khachaturian AS, et al: Reduced risk of Alzheimer disease in users of antioxidant vitamin supplements. Arch Neurol 61:82–88, 2004.

29. Kendell RE: Clinical validity. Psychol Med 19:45–55, 1989.

30. Petersen RC: Clinical evaluation, in Mild Cognitive Impairment: Aging to Alzheimer's Disease. Edited by Petersen RC. New York, Oxford University Press, 2003, pp 229–242.

31. Zaudig M: A new systematic method of measurement and diagnosis of "mild cognitive impairment" and dementia according to ICD-10 and DSM-III-R criteria. Int Psychogeriatr 4 (suppl 2):203–219, 1992.

32. Petersen R: Mild cognitive impairment clinical trials. Nat Rev Drug Discov 2:646–653, 2003.

33. Petersen RC, Thomas RG, Grundman M, et al: Donepezil and vitamin E in the treatment of mild cognitive impairment. N Engl J Med 352:2379–2388, 2005.

34. Aggarwal NT, Wilson RS, Bienias JL, et al: The apolipoprotein E epsilon 4 allele and incident Alzheimer's disease in persons with mild cognitive impairment. Neurocase 11(1):3–7, 2005.

35. Petersen RC, Smith GE, Ivnik RJ, et al: Apolipoprotein E status as a predictor of the development of Alzheimer's disease in memory-impaired individuals. JAMA 273:1274–1278, 1995.

36. Thal LJ, Ferris SH, Kirby L, et al: A randomized, double-blind, study of rofecoxib in patients with mild cognitive impairment. Neuropsychopharmacology 30(6):1204–1215, 2005.

37. Petersen RC, Stevens JC, Ganguli M, et al: Practice parameter: early detection of dementia: mild cognitive impairment (an evidence-based review). Report of the Quality Standards Subcommittee of the American Academy of Neurology. Neurology 56:1133–1142, 2001.

38. Jack CR Jr, Petersen RC, Xu YC, et al: Prediction of AD with MRI-based hippocampal volume in mild cognitive impairment. Neurology 52:1397–1403, 1999.

39. Jack CR Jr, Petersen RC, Xu Y, et al: Rates of hippocampal atrophy correlate with change in clinical status in aging and AD. Neurology 55:484–489, 2000.

40. Jack CR Jr, Petersen RC, Xu YC, et al: Hippocampal atrophy and apolipoprotein E genotype are independently associated with Alzheimer's disease. Ann Neurol 43:303–310, 1998.

41. Kaye JA, Swihart T, Howieson D, et al: Volume loss of the hippocampus and temporal lobe in healthy elderly persons destined to develop dementia. Neurology 48:1297–1304, 1997.

42. Hampel H, Teipel SJ, Fuchsberger T, et al: Value of CSF beta-amyloid1-42 and tau as predictors of Alzheimer's disease in patients with mild cognitive impairment. Mol Psychiatry 9:705–710, 2004.

43. Hampel H, Mitchell A, Blennow K, et al: Core biological marker candidates of Alzheimer's disease—perspectives for diagnosis, prediction of outcome and reflection of biological activity. J Neural Transm 111:247–272, 2004.

44. Klunk WE, Engler H, Nordberg A, et al: Imaging brain amyloid in Alzheimer's disease with Pittsburgh Compound-B. Ann Neurol 55:303–305, 2004.

45. Petersen RC: Focal dementia syndromes: in search of the gold standard. Ann Neurol 49:421–422, 2001.

46. Petersen RC: Mild cognitive impairment: where are we? Alzheimer Dis Assoc Disord 19:166–169, 2005.

5

NEUROPSYCHOLOGICAL TESTING IN THE DIAGNOSIS OF DEMENTIA

Mary Sano, Ph.D.

Although the utility of neuropsychological assessment (NA) in the diagnosis of dementia, a disease characterized by cognitive loss, would seem obvious, early guidelines for assessment of the most common form of dementia, Alzheimer's disease, considered such an evaluation "optional."[1] This may have reflected an era of significant underdetection with initial presentation of obvious symptomatology, frank dementia, and moderate disease. Recent opinions support the value of early detection of subtle cognitive loss, perhaps as a function of public awareness as well as a relatively high cognitive demand brought on by a highly technological and industrial society. Presentation to a medical setting with cognitive complaint is common and a cause of distress for many. In these settings, confirming cognitive loss may not be possible with current screening tools. The presence of extreme age, medical comorbidities, or a variety of social and demographic features may require formal NA to document cognitive deterioration, beyond cognitive complaints. It is apparent that cognitive complaint may not parallel cognitive loss. Recent evidence that subtle or specific cognitive deficits can predict future diagnosis of de-

The author's work is supported by grants AG05138, AG10483, and AG15922.

This chapter is reprinted from Sano M: "Neuropsychological Testing in the Diagnosis of Dementia." *Journal of Geriatric Psychiatry and Neurology* 19:155–159, 2006. Used with permission.

mentia provides additional value to NA, because early detection of risk may permit initiation of treatment and/or disease management at the earliest stage. Also, NA can assist in the characterization of specific dementia diagnoses, which may be important in understanding functional limitations and directing treatment.

It would seem that growing concerns about cognitive health, along with the value of early detection, will increase the importance of NA. There are a range of roles that NA can play in the diagnosis of dementia. Currently available assessment tools for important cognitive domains, such as memory, have shown reasonable clinical utility, but there is a need for better instruments in other domains. Importantly, there is significant potential for NA to contribute to defining the underlying biology of dementia and identifying effective interventions.

Roles for Neuropsychology in Dementia Assessment

Neuropsychological assessment is a valuable tool in the diagnosis of dementia and plays several roles. It can document and confirm cognitive deficits that may be particularly difficult to detect in early stages of the disease and in atypical patient populations. Normative data permit sensitive assessment of very elderly individuals[2] and minority populations as well as individuals with extremes of education.[3] Reports of patients with specific health[4] and disease[5,6] characteristics also add to this knowledge base.

Careful testing across a range of cognitive functions permits the intraindividual examination of patterns of cognitive abilities that can give support to specific diagnostic entities. Even when normative data fail to identify deficits, relative strengths and weaknesses can be identified that may confirm deterioration, identify early disease, and provide clues for the specificity of the dementia.[7]

The presence of comorbid conditions can make diagnostic specificity difficult. Yet several studies demonstrate that tests selected for individuals with specific diagnoses may be able to detect dementia even in compromised populations. Such assessments have been described in stroke,[4] Parkinson's disease,[8] Down syndrome,[8] and others. Although high specificity for one condition over another may be lacking, supportive evidence for contributing diagnoses can be valuable, particularly in designing treatment and management plans in the presence of multiple diagnoses.

Documentation of specific neuropsychological deficits can assist in determining functional consequences. For example, memory deficits may require supervision for compliance with medical management. However, in the absence of other deficits, reminders and mnemonics may be useful. Deficits in executive function, abstract reasoning, and visual-spatial ability increase the likelihood of an impact on a wider range of activities, including driving and handling finances. The evidence for specificity of focal cognitive deficits impairing particular functional abilities is limited. However, there are stronger associations between cognition and function when there are a number of deficits and when they are moderately severe. For example, a combination of memory and processing speed deficits are associated with functional impairment, particularly in complex tasks such as driving and cooking.

Perhaps the strongest support for the value of NA comes from the recent identification of mild cognitive impairment (MCI). This condition was first defined by significant focal memory impairment in the presence of relatively intact cognition in other domains.[10] The presence of this condition has relatively high predictive value for conversion to dementia, specifically Alzheimer's disease. The predictive value and the rate of conversion are highly dependent on NA that permits an evaluation of memory function based on normative data. The ability to identify such a specific population has permitted the design and conducting of successful multiple-center clinical trials, with adequate specification of entry criteria, sample size, and power.[11,12]

Other forms of MCI have been described with nonmemory deficits or multiple domains of impairment short of dementia.[13] Less is known about the predictive utility of other forms,[14] and normative databases for the full range of these cognitive domains are less available, adding to the difficulty of specifying diagnostic criteria.

Finally, NA may provide a method for documenting disease progression. Some reports have suggested that the rate of change in cognitive performance can predict diagnoses up to 10 years later.[15] Others have suggested that cognitive change can be used as an indicator to modify treatment regimens.[16] When complaints occur at early and possibly prodromal stages of disease, the predictive value of NA is particularly important and a comprehensive NA may be needed to determine the type of dementia that is likely to follow. Such an assessment can reveal rate of change, new domains of deficit, and possibly patterns predicting additional etiologies.

Current Strengths of Neuropsychology in Dementia Diagnosis

In the current *Diagnostic and Statistical Manual of Mental Disorders* (DSM) diagnosis for primary progressive dementia, memory impairment is the cornerstone of cognitive impairment.[17] The tools for memory assessment in this domain have been used quite successfully, in part because of norms and standardized assessment and training for administration, scoring, and relatively common interpretation of results. In some cases, tools and scoring have been simplified for use in multiple-center trials, with administration by individuals with minimal expertise. These trends support the idea that NA can be carried out broadly and reliably.

Memory function is sufficiently characterized even to the understanding of the general practitioner. Simple screening tests identify different stages of memory, including registration, working memory, and retention or long-term recall, which is typically assessed by measuring recall after a delay. Our ability to use these constructs in screening tests is based on the availability of normative data. Growing databases of tests for these functions within very elderly patients allow us to characterize the changes associated with aging as well as test performance effects of demographic and clinical variables. This rich database permits the characterization of expected memory performance across a growing age range, through the ninth decade of life.[18,19]

There are general principles on which to interpret performance. Poor recall after a delay is the primary deficit in Alzheimer's disease and can be used to detect the disease early. It is the hallmark of MCI, and the presence of this deficit in the absence of other deficits provides an important marker for the likelihood of further decline to Alzheimer's disease.[10,20] Registration of new information may also permit discrimination among disease entities, particularly when used in combination with other aspects such as recall after a delay. For example, cognitive loss in Parkinson's disease (PD) may be associated with low registration of new items and poor performance on Category Fluency even in the absence of dementia.[8] However, when poor recall after a delay becomes apparent in PD individuals, they are likely to have a concomitant dementia, diagnosed independently of formal testing. Stern and colleagues[8] interpreted this as evidence that dementia is overlaid on this preexisting executive function deficit. A comparison group of patients with Alzheimer's disease performed poorly on delayed recall and on a simpler delayed recognition test, whereas Category Fluency remained relatively high, suggesting a prominent and perhaps specific encoding deficit not as evident in PD.

Because of the growing availability of normative samples from well-characterized patient populations, patterns of deficits have come to have utility in differentiating between diagnostic entities. Other examples include the differentiation of vascular cognitive impairment both from normal performance and from other dementia subtypes. Although not all reports are able to discriminate between these groups, there is evidence of better retrieval in pure vascular dementia than in Alzheimer's disease.[21] Comparing placebo groups in clinical trials with Alzheimer's disease patients alone versus patients with greater vascular components indicates that progression is slower among the latter.[22] Other studies suggest that frontotemporal dementias can be distinguished from Alzheimer's disease based on neuropsychological profiles.[23,24] Like all clinical tests, NA may not guarantee perfect discrimination among diagnoses, but it adds to diagnostic certainty.

Weaknesses of Current Criteria for Diagnosing Dementia

Although there are multiple well-established methods for assessing memory function, assessments for other cognitive areas are less well developed. In the diagnosis of dementia, executive function is often identified as a prominent area of deficit, and the lack of normative data and the limitations of available assessment tools in this area have been widely acknowledged. Despite this, several studies indicate that executive function is distinct from memory and may independently contribute to the disease in predicting both rate of decline and functional impact.[25] Unlike the area of memory function, in which a performance profile has been well characterized for demographic and clinical variables, executive function has limited normative data and few tests with wide application. The lack of tools in this area is highlighted by a recent request for applications from the National Institutes of Health, combining interests of several agencies seeking well-developed instruments to capture relevant executive function across the age span, gender, and other demographic and cultural factors, with special attention to create tools for the detection of this cognitive deficit in a range of disease entities.[26]

An additional limitation of current diagnostic criteria is the focus on cognitive impairment while ignoring complaint. Perhaps this omission in the current criteria is made on the basis of low correlation between cognitive complaint and neuropsychological testing.[27] In fact, complaint is likely to be associated with other diagnostic entities and demographic features.[28] Yet, several studies indicate that complaint may be an early marker of deteriorating cognition, perhaps in cognitive domains and testing settings where current normative data are not sufficiently sensitive to capture subtle change. For example, in community-based studies the "new onset" of memory complaint was associated with the subsequent deterioration in cognitive score.[29] Additionally, the absence of complaint by self or other raises the question of how meaningful the entity is.[30]

Because cognitive complaint is distressing and can be persistent, it would seem worthy of inclusion in the diagnostic criteria, which would permit evaluation and treatment of this symptom alone. Research diagnoses that focus on lesser syndromes include several that focus on complaint. Age-associated memory impairment reflects a condition of complaint with age-appropriate memory performance. Age-related (or age-associated) cognitive decline includes complaint with any type of cognitive performance below age norm and MCI, which includes memory complaint[10,13] acknowledged by self or other with significant deficit, usually in memory and possibly other areas. Currently, the DSM criteria do not acknowledge these conditions, limiting health care interest and resource to these entities.

Another related area that requires improvement is methodology to fully characterize impairment in social and occupational functioning. Both inventory and performance-based measures are available and are able to demonstrate deficits in the presence of frank dementia. Like cognitive function, social and occupational functioning may require age-based norms as well as norms for other demographic features, including gender and education. Tools to identify deficits in social and occupational function in mild forms of cognitive impairment are poorly developed and not predictive of decline.[31] Measures of functional ability are most sensitive in dementia when the clinical report is provided by someone other than the patient, but this is not the case in the presence of MCI. Some studies suggest that self-reports are at least as sensitive to change as informant report,[32] whereas others report discrepancies in self- and other evaluations of activities of daily living.[33] Subtle cognitive changes are not well correlated with most measures of functional impairment, although several reports indicate that memory and executive function deficit may predict later functional decline.[34,35] Within executive function, sequencing and planning appear to be more predictive of functional loss than cognitive speed.[24]

Promising Hypotheses for Future Research

One of the most prominent areas of research is the identification of potential biological therapies for dementia. For Alzheimer's disease, the most common dementia, the perceived underlying etiology has been the focus for interventions. All currently approved treatments have used cognitive outcomes to demonstrate efficacy. Models for the reduction of amyloid and the minimization of protein aggregation to form plaques are widely being investigated. Therapeutic development focused on tau reduction is also perceived as a creative and viable approach that may address a range of dementias. These studies have used global neuropsychological outcomes as primary outcome measures. However, as we grow sensitive to mild and specific cognitive loss, which may have important functional significance, it becomes reasonable to consider the biological basis of these early symptoms and perhaps address the pharmacological basis of symptom reduction. There are increasing data to suggest a genetic influence on specific cognitive function. For example, Small and colleagues[36] demonstrated that among nondemented elderly patients, the presence of the *APOE* ε4 allele was associated with a small but robust difference in memory testing but not in a global measure of cognition. This effect was reduced with age. Others have shown this allele to be associated with reduced hippocampal volume in nondemented individuals, with the most pronounced effect before age 65.[37] Change in other cognitive domains may also have specific genetic influences. Heritability studies among twins demonstrate that accelerating changes in executive function (specifically, deterioration in processing speed rather than memory or visual-spatial skills) share genetic variance.[38] These findings may provide hints to the biology of interventions that would reduce deterioration of specific cognitive function.

An alternative approach to therapeutics is to consider if specific cognitive deficits should be the target of intervention. Because many genetic influences are reduced with age, and impairing cognitive loss will occur in the very old long before the identification of dementia pathology, perhaps focusing on pharmacology to enhance specific cognitive function, such as memory, attention, or executive function, is a reasonable approach for the future. Mechanisms for specific interventions can be identified for several cognitive domains. Age-related losses of striatal dopamine transporter density have been associated with age-related deficits in episodic memory and executive functioning in nondemented elderly people.[39] Dopaminergic agonists appear to improve working memory in older nondemented adults, suggesting the possibility that specific cognitive functions can be modulated.[40] Pharmacological increase in cholinergic neurotransmission has been demonstrated to specifically improve hippocampal function in imaging studies[41] and memory function in clinical trials.[42] These studies highlight the possibility that focal cognitive deficits that may be clinically compromising are potentially amenable to pharmacological intervention. NA provides the tools to make these important distinctions.

Conclusion

Neuropsychological assessment offers a valuable tool for diagnosing dementia and possibly for predicting the clinical course. Additionally, neuropsychology offers the ability to detect subtle cognitive change that can be the source of significant distress. Currently, detection of deficits in memory is particularly sensitive because of relatively broad and robust normative data through extreme age ranges. As this normative database grows for tools to assess other cognitive areas, such as executive function, visual-spatial ability, and attention, sensitive evaluation in these areas can also be achieved. Given growing cognitive demands to accomplish routine daily activities, even subtle complaints may be important to identify, because they may have significant yet unrecognized impact on function.

NA has played a major role in identifying treatments for dementia, and new approaches to Alzheimer's disease therapy that focus on the underlying etiology will continue to use cognitive testing as the primary outcome measure. As the ability to reliably measure specific domains improves, neuropsychological tools may provide an opportunity to identify treatments for a range of focal cognitive deficits.

References

1. Knopman DS, DeKosky ST, Cummings JL, et al: Practice parameter: diagnosis of dementia (an evidence-based review). Report of the Quality Standards Subcommittee of the American Academy of Neurology. Neurology 56:1143–1153, 2001.
2. Ivnik R, Malec J, Smith G, et al: Mayo's Older Americans Normative Studies: WMS-R norms for ages 56 to 97. Clin Neuropsychol 6(suppl):49–82, 1992.
3. Stricks L, Pittman J, Jacobs DM, et al: Normative data for a brief neuropsychological battery administered to English- and Spanish-speaking community-dwelling elders. J Int Neuropsychol Soc 4:311–318, 1998.
4. Desmond DW, Tatemichi TK, Paik M, et al: Risk factors for cerebrovascular disease as correlates of cognitive function in a stroke-free cohort. Arch Neurol 50:162–166, 1993.
5. Tatemichi TK, Desmond DW, Stern Y, et al: Cognitive impairment after stroke: frequency, patterns, and relationship to functional abilities. J Neurol Neurosurg Psychiatry 57:202–207, 1994.

6. Kieburtz K, McDermott M, Como P, et al: The effect of deprenyl and tocopherol on cognitive performance in early untreated Parkinson's disease. Parkinson Study Group. Neurology 44:1756–1759, 1994.

7. de Mendonca A, Ribeiro F, Guerreiro M, et al: Frontotemporal mild cognitive impairment. J Alzheimers Dis 6:1–9, 2004.

8. Stern Y, Richards M, Sano M, et al: Comparison of cognitive changes in patients with Alzheimer's and Parkinson's disease. Arch Neurol 50:1040–1045, 1993.

9. Sano M, Aisen PS, Dalton AJ, et al: Assessment of aging individuals with Down syndrome in clinical trials: results of baseline measures. Journal of Policy and Practice in Intellectual Disabilities 2:126–138, 2005.

10. Petersen CP, Doody R, Kurz A, et al: Current concepts in mild cognitive impairment. Arch Neurol 58:1985–1992, 2001.

11. Levy R. Aging-associated cognitive decline. Int Psychogeriatr 6:63–68, 1994.

12. Grundman M, Petersen RC, Ferris SH, et al: Alzheimer's Disease Cooperative Study. Mild cognitive impairment can be distinguished from Alzheimer disease and normal aging for clinical trials. Arch Neurol 61:59–66, 2004.

13. Salloway S, Ferris S, Kluger A, et al: Donepezil 401 Study Group. Efficacy of donepezil in mild cognitive impairment: a randomized placebo-controlled trial. Neurology 63:651–657, 2004.

14. Lopez OL, Jagust WJ, Dulberg C, et al: Risk factors for mild cognitive impairment in the Cardiovascular Health Study Cognition Study, Part 2. Arch Neurol 60:1394–1399, 2003.

15. Tierney MC, Yao C, Kiss A, et al: Neuropsychological tests accurately predict incident Alzheimer disease after 5 and 10 years. Neurology 64:1853–1859, 2005.

16. Doody RS, Dunn JK, Huang E, et al: A method for estimating duration of illness in Alzheimer's disease. Dement Geriatr Cogn Disord 17:1–4, 2004.

17. American Psychiatric Association: Diagnostic and Statistical Manual of Mental Disorders, 4th Edition, Text Revision. Washington, DC, American Psychiatric Association, 2000.

18. Welsh KA, Butters N, Hughes JP, et al: Detection and staging of dementia in Alzheimer's disease. Use of the neuropsychological measures developed for the Consortium to Establish a Registry for Alzheimer's Disease. Arch Neurol 49:448–452, 1992.

19. Beeri MS, Schmeidler J, Sano M, et al: Age, gender, and education norms on the CERAD neuropsychological battery in the oldest old. Neurology 67:1006–1010, 2006.

20. Graham NL, Emery T, Hodges JR: Distinctive cognitive profiles in Alzheimer's disease and subcortical vascular dementia. J Neurol Neurosurg Psychiatry 75:61–71, 2004.

21. Traykov L, Baudic S, Raoux N, et al: Patterns of memory impairment and perseverative behavior discriminate early Alzheimer's disease from subcortical vascular dementia. J Neurol Sci 229–230:75–79, 2005.

22. Erkinjuntti T, Kurz A, Gauthier S, et al: Efficacy of galantamine in probable vascular dementia and Alzheimer's disease combined with cerebrovascular disease: a randomised trial. Lancet 359:1283–1290, 2002.

23. Srikanth S, Nagaraja AV, Ratnavalli E: Neuropsychiatric symptoms in dementia-frequency, relationship to dementia severity and comparison in Alzheimer's disease, vascular dementia and frontotemporal dementia. J Neurol Sci 236:43–48, 2005.

24. Thompson JC, Stopford CL, Snowden JS, et al: Qualitative neuropsychological performance characteristics in frontotemporal dementia and Alzheimer's disease. J Neurol Neurosurg Psychiatry 76:920–927, 2005.

25. Rapp MA, Schnaider Beeri M, Schmeidler J, et al: Relationship of neuropsychological performance to functional status in nursing home residents and community-dwelling older adults. Am J Geriatr Psychiatry 13:450–459, 2005.

26. RFP NIH-NINDS-05-02. Domain Specific Tasks of Executive Function in Neurological Disorders. Notice no. NOT-NS-05-006. Available at: http://www.ninds.nih.gov/. Release date 4/1/2005. Accessed on July 21, 2005.

27. Purser JL, Fillenbaum GG, Wallace RB: Memory complaint is not necessary for diagnosis of mild cognitive impairment and does not predict 10-year trajectories of functional disability, word recall, or Short Portable Mental Status Questionnaire limitations. J Am Geriatr Soc 54:335–338, 2006.

28. Kliegel M, Zimprich D, Eschen A: What do subjective cognitive complaints in persons with aging-associated cognitive decline reflect? Int Psychogeriatr 17:499–512, 2005.

29. Schofield PW, Marder K, Dooneief G, et al: Association of subjective memory complaints with subsequent cognitive decline in community-dwelling elderly individuals with baseline cognitive impairment. Am J Psychiatry 154:609–615, 1997.

30. Royal DR: Mild cognitive impairment and functional status. J Am Geriatr Soc 54:163–165, 2006.

31. Nygard L: Instrumental activities of daily living: a stepping-stone towards Alzheimer's disease diagnosis in subjects with mild cognitive impairment? Acta Neurol Scand Suppl 179:42–46, 2003.

32. Farias ST, Mungas D, Jagust W: Degree of discrepancy between self and other-reported everyday functioning by cognitive status: dementia, mild cognitive impairment, and healthy elders. Int J Geriatr Psychiatry 20:827–834, 2005.

33. Albert SM, Michaels K, Padilla M, et al: Functional significance of mild cognitive impairment in elderly patients without a dementia diagnosis. Am J Geriatr Psychiatry 7:213–220, 1999.

34. Tuokko H, Morris C, Ebert P: Mild cognitive impairment and everyday functioning in older adults. Neurocase 11:40–47, 2005.

35. Royal DR: Mild cognitive impairment and functional status. J Am Geriatr Soc 54:163–165, 2006.

36. Small BJ, Rosnick CB, Fratiglioni L, et al: Apolipoprotein E and cognitive performance: a meta-analysis. Psychol Aging 19:592–600, 2004.

37. Lind J, Larsson A, Persson J, et al: Reduced hippocampal volume in non-demented carriers of the apolipoprotein E epsilon4: relation to chronological age and recognition memory. Neurosci Lett 396:23–27, 2006.

38. Finkel D, Reynolds CA, McArdle JJ, et al: The longitudinal relationship between processing speed and cognitive ability: genetic and environmental influences. Behav Genet 35:535–549, 2005.

39. Erixon-Lindroth N, Farde L, Wahlin TB, et al: The role of the striatal dopamine transporter in cognitive aging. Psychiatry Res 138:1–12, 2005.

40. Peretti CS, Gierski F, Harrois S: Cognitive skill learning in healthy older adults after 2 months of double-blind treatment with piribedil. Psychopharmacology (Berl) 176:175–181, 2004.

41. Gron G, Brandenburg I, Wunderlich AP, et al: Inhibition of hippocampal function in mild cognitive impairment: targeting the cholinergic hypothesis. Neurobiol Aging 27:78–87, 2006.

42. Petersen RC, Thomas RG, Grundman M, et al: Alzheimer's Disease Cooperative Study Group. Vitamin E and donepezil for the treatment of mild cognitive impairment. N Engl J Med 352:2379–2388, 2005.

6

DIAGNOSTIC CATEGORIES AND CRITERIA FOR NEUROPSYCHIATRIC SYNDROMES IN DEMENTIA

Research Agenda for DSM-V

Dilip V. Jeste, M.D.
Thomas W. Meeks, M.D.
Daniel S. Kim, M.D.
George S. Zubenko, M.D., Ph.D.

Psychiatric symptoms, such as psychosis and depression, were recognized as important aspects of dementia beginning with the case of Augustine D. described by Alzheimer in 1907. Despite this observation, focus over the past century has often centered narrowly on impairments of memory and other cognitive domains that

This work was supported in part by grants MH19934-13 (Dr. Jeste) and MH47346 (Dr. Zubenko) from the National Institute of Mental Health, and by the Department of Veterans Affairs.

This chapter is reprinted from Jeste DV, Meeks TW, Kim DS, et al.: "Research Agenda for DSM-V: Diagnostic Categories and Criteria for Neuropsychiatric Syndromes in Dementia." *Journal of Geriatric Psychiatry and Neurology* 19:160–171, 2006. Used with permission.

have been used to define the clinical syndrome of dementia. The high prevalence and clinical significance of other psychiatric disturbances in dementia are now receiving increasing attention. Most estimates of the prevalence of neuropsychiatric signs and symptoms in dementia range from 60% to 80%.[1] In addition to causing considerable patient suffering, neuropsychiatric symptoms are linked to the development of depressive disorders and general distress among caregivers and increase the rate of institutionalization of patients with dementia.[2] Institutionalization exacts a high emotional toll on patients and families as well as a high economic toll on the health care system. Economic analysis has demonstrated that 30% of the cost of dementia-related health care of patients with Alzheimer's disease (AD) is directly attributable to the management of psychiatric symptoms.[2]

Given the impact of psychiatric symptoms in dementia, it is important that diagnostic descriptions of dementia include and coherently organize these symptoms. This task requires the establishment of clear definitions of psychiatric signs and symptoms that can be reliably identified using operationalized diagnostic criteria. The latter task requires special attention to the evaluation of patients whose dementia may interfere with their ability to accurately report their experiences. On the basis of subsequent empirical research using these prerequisites, identifiable symptom clusters are emerging that appear to have clinical utility, including characteristic family and natural histories, treatment responses, and shared biological underpinnings (syndromes). This progress should continue to be reflected in the evolution of the *Diagnostic and Statistical Manual of Mental Disorders* (DSM).

Psychiatric complications of dementia were first included as a group of identical subtypes of "primary degenerative dementia and multi-infarct dementia" in DSM-III.[3] These subtypes included "with delirium," "with delusions," "with depression," and "uncomplicated." In DSM-III-R,[4] the diagnosis "primary degenerative dementia" was converted to "primary degenerative dementia of the Alzheimer's type" (PDD-AT), with modest diagnostic clarifications that were tailored to this specific dementia. However, DSM-III-R included no revisions of the psychiatric subtypes for either PDD-AT or multi-infarct dementia. In both DSM-III and DSM-III-R, the subtypes of delusions and depression were conceptualized as clinical "features," without further clarification, whereas delirium was characterized as a syndrome with explicit diagnostic inclusion and exclusion criteria.

In DSM-III and DSM-III-R, dementias were included in the section called "Organic Mental Syndromes and Disorders." This section terminology was abandoned in DSM-IV because the term *organic mental disorder* incorrectly implies that "nonorganic" mental disorders do not have a biological basis. DSM-IV placed more emphasis on core cognitive deficits in the diagnosis of dementia than its predecessors, because personality change was excluded from the diagnostic criteria for this disorder regardless of etiology. Dementia of the Alzheimer's type (DAT) was substituted for PDD-AT, and "vascular dementia" was substituted for "multi-infarct dementia" in DSM-III-R, with minor clarifications of the diagnostic criteria for both.

DSM-IV introduced a new subtype of DAT to identify cases with early (≤65 years) or late (>65 years) symptomatic onset of cognitive impairment. Consistent with its predecessors, DSM-IV included identical psychiatric subtypes of both DAT and vascular dementia: "with delirium," "with delusions," "with depressed mood," and "uncomplicated." In contrast to DSM-III and DSM-III-R, the subtypes other than delirium required that the corresponding psychiatric complication be the "predominant feature," a noteworthy change that would favor underreporting less prominent or concurrent psychiatric disturbances. As with its predecessors, there was also no means to distinguish patients who developed depressed mood from those who met full symptom criteria for a major depressive episode or to identify patients who experienced hallucinations in the context of dementia. The specifier "with behavioral disturbance" was introduced in DSM-IV to note clinically significant behavioral disturbances in addition to the psychiatric subtypes, but this addition was not fully integrated into the diagnoses and could not be coded.

Growing recognition of the importance of psychiatric disturbances that occur in the context of dementias has been reflected in efforts to properly incorporate them within DSM-III, DSM-III-R, and DSM-IV. However, a large and growing body of clinical evidence has highlighted areas where improvement seems warranted. Clear, practical criteria for describing the psychiatric disturbances of dementia have generally been lacking. The rationale for including an "uncomplicated" subtype, used to simply denote the absence of delirium, depression, or delusions, is unclear and misleading. At best it is redundant, because each of the other subtypes was coded independently in DSM-III to DSM-IV. Furthermore, dementia is often complicated by clinically significant psychiatric disturbances other than delirium, depression, or delusions. Finally, even in the absence of psychiatric ("noncognitive") disturbances, few would characterize progressive dementia as "uncomplicated." Except for the "with behavioral disturbance" descriptor that was not fully integrated into the dementia classifications of DSM-IV, the ability to capture the range of clinically important observable behavioral disturbances (e.g., wandering, assaultiveness, sleep disturbance) and other psychiatric disturbances (e.g., hallucinations) is inadequate. Ambiguity also remains in whether to describe particular psychiatric disturbances of patients with DAT using available psychiatric subtypes or as separate Axis I diagnoses (e.g., delirium, psychiatric condition attributable to AD, mood disorder not otherwise specified).

DSM-IV-TR: A Step in the Right Direction

Most recently, DSM-IV-TR[6] embodied a reorganized classification of the psychiatric disturbances of the dementias that addresses a number of the weaknesses of its predecessors. Changes have focused on DAT, where the preponderance of empirical evidence in this area has accumulated. Fewer studies have addressed the psychiatric disturbances in vascular and other dementias, and DSM-IV-TR remains unchanged from DSM-IV and the *International Classification of Diseases,* 9th Revision (ICD-9) in these areas.

In DSM-IV-TR, DAT retains the same early-/late-onset subtypes as in DSM-IV, although the current coding system depends exclusively on the presence/absence of a clinically significant behavioral disturbance. The use of this binary coding has the potential to readily identify cases for which there is a clinically significant psychiatric disturbance. Guidance on whether "behavioral" is meant to apply to psychiatric disturbances generally (signs and symptoms) or only those that are observable is not provided. However, this approach has the benefit of highlighting the presence of clinically significant disturbances, regardless of their specific content, while eliminating the "uncomplicated" subtype.

Other prominent clinical features related to DAT are indicated by coding the specific additional mental disorders attributable to AD on Axis I. This approach has several advantages over those adopted by DSM-III to DSM-IV. It provides clarity on the specific approach to use for diagnostic formulation and coding that was ambiguous in previous editions. For the first time, the psychiatric manifestations attributable to AD are described as such, rather than simply as associated features, an important conceptual change that is consistent with empirical research findings. Furthermore, the recording procedures embrace the use of "psychotic disorder" (delusions and/or hallucinations), and "mood disorder" (with depressive features, major depressive-like episode, manic features, mixed features) attributable to AD, an approach that is also supported by substantial empirical evidence.

Recent Efforts to Refine Classification

Efforts have been made in recent years to address the problem of classifying psychiatric disturbances in dementia. For instance, in 1996 the International Psychogeriatric Association labeled these neuropsychiatric symptoms as "behavioral and psychological symptoms of dementia (BPSD)."[7] These were defined as "signs and symptoms of disturbed perception, thought content, mood, or behavior that frequently occur in patients with dementia." This provided a unifying concept for the field and helped to focus attention on neuropsychiatric symptoms in dementia. Yet the concept of BPSD is too broad as a diagnostic category. With this realization, attention began to focus on defining important subtypes within BPSD.

Current diagnostic groupings in psychiatry are predominantly developed on the basis of similar clinical phenotypes. Emerging diagnostic constructs for neuropsychiatric syndromes in dementia are drawn from and have theoretical congruence with nondementia diagnoses in psychiatry (e.g., psychotic disorders, mood disorders). As in medicine generally, the goal for diagnostic categorization would ultimately lie in groupings based on shared etiology. In this regard, significant progress has been made in studies of the neurobiological underpinnings of psychosis and depression in AD. Yet the promise of genetics and neuroimaging for improving diagnostic specificity in the neuropsychiatric syndromes of dementia still remains unfulfilled.

One approach to categorizing neuropsychiatric symptoms has included cross-sectional analyses of how various symptoms cluster together.[8] Using factor analysis, one study reported the most robust psychiatric symptom groupings among persons with dementia to be agitation, affective disturbance, and altered circadian rhythms.[9] Yet another similar study in Alzheimer's dementia found groupings of agitation/anxiety, psychosis, aggression, depression, and activity disturbance/wandering.[10,11] It demonstrated that co-occurrence of various psychiatric symptoms in dementia is the rule rather than an exception, and it demonstrated clinically significant behavioral disturbances even among patients with AD classified as "uncomplicated" according to past DSM nomenclature. Lyketsos and colleagues[12] found three "classes" of symptoms among patients with AD: asymptomatic or monosymptomatic patients, polysymptomatic patients with prominent affective disturbance, and polysymptomatic patients with prominent psychotic disturbance. Although comorbidity is common among neuropsychiatric syndromes in dementia, this is not unlike the epidemiological data observed in other psychotic, mood, and anxiety disorders; construct validity remains a prominent challenge for psychiatry as a whole.

Despite these attempts, diagnostic categories must be based on more than the co-occurrence of symptoms. Neuropsychiatric syndromes must be organized in a way that allows systematic examination of reliability and validity and that takes into account natural course, prognosis, and treatment response. Early efforts to address this goal in AD revealed that operationalized criteria could reliably assign patients to the diagnostic subgroupings used in DSM-III-R (with delirium, with delusions, with depression, and uncomplicated). Additionally, each behavioral subtype responded longitudinally to targeted treatments based on the predominant symptoms.[11] Yet there remained heterogeneity in how researchers and clinicians described the psychiatric complications of dementia. The existing diagnostic categories in DSM still failed to capture the full spectrum of neuropsychiatric symptoms. To address this issue, separate consensus groups were convened to develop provisional diagnostic criteria for three commonly recognized neuropsychiatric syndromes observed in AD: psychosis, depression, and sleep disturbance.[13–15] These proposed criteria are based on at least some research and clinical experience, giving them good face validity. Yet additional work is needed to validate these diagnoses further. Any proposed criteria at this juncture are likely to (indeed should) elicit debate.

Acknowledging the need for this debate, we will review four of the most commonly researched categories of psychiatric symptoms in AD: psychosis, depression, agitation, and sleep disturbance. These constructs are a work in progress but represent the diagnostic categories most likely to be sufficiently validated for inclusion in the next revision of DSM. However, this by no means implies that these four categories alone encompass the full range of psychiatric symptoms seen in dementia or that they are completely independent of one another. Other important symptoms have been identified, including apathy, anxiety, and disinhibition; further research in these areas also seems warranted. Likewise, although vascular dementia and dementia with Lewy bodies are common and appear to have many neuropsychiatric symptoms similar to AD, the bulk of the evidence available is in AD. Existing data in these other dementias will be briefly discussed in the context of each syndrome.

Specific Neuropsychiatric Syndromes

PSYCHOSIS OF ALZHEIMER'S DISEASE

Epidemiology

Psychotic symptoms in AD typically consist of delusions and/or hallucinations. Although certain aspects of hallucinations and delusions may differ (e.g., comorbid symptoms, risk factors, brain regions implicated), they are most often classified together. The prevalence of psychosis is quite substantial, with estimates for delusions in AD ranging from 9.3% to 63% (median=36%) and estimates for hallucinations ranging from 4% to 41% (median=18%).[16] The wide variability in results stems, in part, from methodological inconsistencies, such as different diagnostic criteria for dementia and psychosis across studies. Several clinical risk factors for developing psychosis in dementia have been identified, including severity of cognitive impairment, African American ethnicity, and possibly lower educational level, extrapyramidal symptoms, and sensory impairments.[16,17] The consequences of psychosis of AD include higher caregiver distress, institutionalization rates, and rates of functional decline.[16]

Evidence for a Distinct Syndrome

As mentioned above, psychosis proved to be a coherent grouping of psychiatric symptoms in AD in studies using cluster and factor analysis.[10–12] Additionally, the psychosis of AD appears different from primary psychotic disorders, such as schizophrenia, in important ways. Disorganized speech, disorganized behavior, and negative symptoms characteristic of schizophrenia have not proved useful concepts in describing the psychosis of AD. Delusions in AD often involve theft, abandonment, or misidentification. The delusions are also typically less complex and organized than those observed in schizophrenia. Likewise, hallucinatory experiences in AD are often distinct from those observed in schizophrenia. Visual hallucinations predominate, in lieu of the auditory hallucinations characteristic of schizophrenia.

The psychotic symptoms seen in AD have a more variable course than those in schizophrenia and respond to lower doses of antipsychotic medications.[13]

Etiology

AD with psychosis also appears distinct from AD without psychosis in various biological studies. Efforts to characterize the neurobiology underlying the psychosis of AD have implicated frontal lobe involvement in neuropsychological studies.[18] Postmortem studies have revealed increased frontal and temporal β-amyloid and neurofibrillary tangles and changes in hippocampal neuronal counts compared with AD without psychosis.[19,20] These observations are consistent with the increase in the rate of cognitive decline experienced by AD patients with psychosis.[21] Neurochemical studies of postmortem brain tissue have also revealed changes in cortical and subcortical levels of amine neurotransmitters, including relative preservation of dopamine in the substantia nigra and reduction of serotonin in the hippocampus.[19] However, no neuropathological or neurochemical changes could be considered pathognomonic for psychosis of AD in individual patients. Genes that have been implicated in psychosis of AD include those for dopamine$_3$ and serotonin$_{2A}$ receptors.[22] There is also some evidence that the *APOE* ε4 allele is associated with the development of psychosis in AD.[22] Electroencephalography has also been used as a probe for biological correlates of psychosis in AD, with some findings of increased δθ activity in psychosis.[23] Neuroimaging results suggest decreased frontal and temporal lobe functioning and/or volume.[24,25]

Proposed Criteria

Drawing on expert opinion synthesizing many of the data summarized above, Jeste and Finkel[13] in 2000 proposed provisional diagnostic criteria for the psychosis of AD. Important features of these criteria include duration and time-of-onset criteria, a requirement for functional impairment, and important exclusionary etiologies. As mentioned before, these criteria will serve as a useful model for testing diagnostic validity and reliability and ultimately for standardizing clinical studies of the epidemiology, neurobiology, and treatment of psychosis in AD. Already, early evidence supports that there is good interrater and test–retest reliability for these proposed criteria.[22]

Treatment

Antipsychotics have been the logical treatment of choice for psychosis of AD, beginning with first-generation, or "typical," antipsychotics, especially haloperidol. With the advent of second-generation, or "atypical," antipsychotics, better side-effect profiles were presumed, and this ushered in the use of this class. Overall, antipsychotics appear to have modest efficacy for treating the psychosis of AD.[26] Although there is good evidence indicating that movement disorders in particular are less common with second-generation agents,[27] debate about their overall superiority in safety has grown with recent Food and Drug Administration warnings for the use of second-generation antipsychotics in dementia.[28] Results are forthcoming from the large, National Institutes of Health–sponsored, multiple-center clinical trial (CATIE-AD), which randomly assigned AD patients with psychosis and/or agitation to treatment with risperidone, olanzapine, quetiapine, or citalopram.[29]

Non-Alzheimer's Dementias

Although the evidence concerning psychosis in other types of dementia is notably scarcer than for AD, certain similarities and differences are known. For instance, visual hallucinations are part of the core diagnostic construct of dementia with Lewy bodies, occurring in up to 77% of patients. Delusions are also quite common, with a reported prevalence of 46%.[30] Vascular dementia may be somewhat less prone than AD or dementia with Lewy bodies to cause delusional symptoms, although not all studies have verified this. Psychosis remains relatively common among patients with vascular dementia, with one study reporting the prevalence to be as high as 46% among hospitalized patients.[31] Psychosis in frontotemporal dementia is even less characterized, although at least one study found a prevalence of psychotic symptoms similar to that in AD.[32]

DEPRESSION OF ALZHEIMER'S DISEASE

Epidemiology

Clinically significant depression is a common and important complication of AD that increases the suffering of patients and their families, produces excess disability, promotes institutionalization, and hastens death.[33] As with psychosis, the reported prevalence estimates of depression in dementia have been quite variable, attributable in part to differing definitions of depression across studies. Estimates of the point prevalence of depression symptoms in AD have been as high as 86%.[34] In clinical samples, estimates of syndromal depression in AD range from 15% to 25%, whereas an additional 20%–30% of patients may have subsyndromal depression symptoms.[35] The relapsing–remitting nature of depression in AD suggests that an even larger proportion of patients eventually experience a major depressive episode before death.[11] A recent report using prospective data and a structured diagnostic interview (Clinical Assessment of Depression in Dementia) developed for reliably diagnosing depressive episodes in AD found this diagnosis in 35% of those with probable AD.[36]

Reported risk factors for depression in AD include family history of a mood disorder, personal history of a mood disorder, female gender, and early-onset dementia.[36,37] The natural course of depression in dementia has not been systematically characterized, but available evidence suggests a recurrent or chronic course. The persistence of depressive symptoms in AD at 6 months was reported as 30%–40% in one study.[35] Some studies suggest that depression is more common in mild to moderate stages of AD, although there is speculation this may be an artifact of reduced ability to express depressed mood verbally in more cognitively impaired patients.[35] Depression may even precede and serve as a prodrome to the eventual development of AD. There is some debate as to whether depression may be a risk factor for AD as well.[37] In a recent family study of recurrent early-onset major depressive disorder (MDD), a severe and strongly familial form of MDD, the age-specific prevalence of AD-like dementia among extended relatives was more than twice that reported for the general population.[38]

Evidence for a Distinct Syndrome

Several characteristics of depression in AD appear to distinguish it from depression in elderly patients with normal cognition. For instance, the previously summarized prevalence estimates of depression in AD are considerably higher than the 1.4% figure reported for community-dwelling nondemented elders by the Epidemiologic Catchment Area study.[39] Furthermore, the clinical presentations of major depressive episodes (MDEs) among AD patients have been reported to differ in meaningful ways from those experienced by nondemented elders.[36] Despite some symptom overlap, patients with AD have reported more concentration difficulties and indecisiveness and less sleep disturbance and feelings of worthlessness or guilt during depressive episodes. There is some evidence that the symptoms fluctuate more in depression of AD than in MDD. Overall the symptom severity of depression in AD may be less than that observed in major depression among nondemented elders, consistent with reduced rates of suicidality reported in some studies of AD-associated depression.[14,36,40]

Most[38,41,42] but not all[43] studies have reported that a family history of MDD was significantly higher among first-degree relatives of AD patients with depression than in those who did not develop this behavioral complication. This suggests that the development of depression in AD may rely on an interaction of specific degenerative events with one or more familial factors that confer vulnerability to the development of this mood disorder. This again distinguishes depression in AD from late-onset MDD in elders with normal cognition, which is rarely familial. As described below, depression of AD has also been validated by postmortem studies that differentiate this behavioral syndrome from AD without depression, AD with psychosis, and normal aging.

As with all psychiatric symptoms in AD, depressed mood often co-occurs with other psychiatric symptoms, and major depression in AD exhibits some features that appear to overlap with other psychiatric syndromes. This emphasizes the importance of relying on syndromes rather than individual symptoms when characterizing psychiatric complications in AD. For instance, depression and apathy may appear similar in some respects among AD patients. Apathy and depression scores were correlated in some studies, and apathy overlaps conceptually with the anhedonia characteristic of depression. There is reason to believe, however, that depressed mood and apathy may be the predominant manifestations of distinguishable brain abnormalities, as argued in a recent review.[44] Different brain regions were abnormal in a functional neuroimaging study that compared AD patients categorized as depressed versus apathetic.[45]

Not surprisingly, comorbidity of depression in AD with several other behavioral syndromes has been reported. Depression in AD increased the odds of having delusions by a factor of 6.8 in one sample, although depression seemed less related to hallucinations.[46] Depression may also increase the odds of agitation in patients with dementia.[47] Other comorbid symptoms may include anxiety and mood lability, and the latter may overlap with irritability in some patients. Despite these complexities, major depression is among the most valid neuropsychiatric constructs in AD and has repeatedly emerged as a distinct symptom cluster in studies to date.[9,10,12] The neurobiology of major depression associated with AD is outlined below and implicates some pathology that appears distinct from that of AD without major depression as well as from major depression without AD.

Etiology

The causes of depression in AD have been investigated from several angles. Most studies show no direct association between patient insight into disability or illness and the development of depression in AD.[48] The "psychological" reaction to the illness could still be an important factor for certain patients, but biological factors likely contribute more significantly to the depressive symptoms in AD.

Clinicopathological studies indicate that the emergence of major depression in AD is associated with selective loss of noradrenergic cells in the locus coeruleus, along with some evidence for degeneration of dopaminergic neurons in the substantia nigra and serotonergic cells in the dorsal raphe nuclei and relative preservation of cholinergic neurons in the nucleus basalis.[49–52] These degenerative changes appear to involve apoptotic events in the brainstem.[33] Consistent with these observations, dementia patients with major depression have been reported to manifest significant reductions of norepinephrine in the cortex and modest reductions in serotonin in projection areas of the dorsal raphe nuclei.[53] Initial reports produced divergent findings regarding the association of the *APOE* ε4 allele with late-onset MDD,[54,55] although subsequent studies have not supported this association,[56] which contrasts with the somewhat more consistent association between *APOE* ε4 and psychosis of AD. Functional neuroimaging findings have found frontal lobe hypometabolism in depressed AD patients.[57] Positron emission tomography studies have also revealed distinct findings for symptoms of depression and psychosis in AD. Depression scores correlated with hypometabolism in the frontal lobe, whereas delusions were associated with increased metabolism in the inferior temporal gyrus and decreased metabolism in the occipital lobe.[58]

Proposed Criteria

As with psychosis, a consensus group convened to develop provisional criteria for depression of AD.[14] The criteria were derived from those of major depression but were modified according to empirical evidence and expert opinion of how major depression in AD differs. In some ways these criteria are more inclusive than those of major depression. Examples of pertinent changes are 1) requiring three instead of five symptoms; 2) not requiring that depressive symptoms be present nearly every day; 3) including criteria for irritability and social isolation/withdrawal; and 4) modifying the criterion of loss of interest/pleasure to include the perception of decreased positive affect in response to social contacts or usually pleasurable activities. Unique specifiers can be applied that describe comorbid symptoms, depression history, and time course.

Others have argued that these criteria are overly inclusive and that the DSM-IV-TR concepts of major depression and minor depression have validity in AD.[36,59] Several studies described earlier in this section, including clinical, neuropathological, and neurochemical studies, used the syndromal diagnosis of major depression in AD. Structured diagnostic interviews have been validated for diagnosing major depression in AD as well.[36] These methods use an inclusive approach to diagnosing major depression, in which presumed etiology for any individual diagnostic criterion does not need to be evaluated in order to count toward a diagnosis. This stands in contrast to the consensus-proposed criteria for depression of AD, which "do not include symptoms that … are clearly due to a medical condition other than Alzheimer's disease, or are a direct result of non–mood-related dementia symptoms."[14] Direct comparisons of the merits of these differing diagnostic constructs will help clarify which construct provides the most diagnostic reliability and validity.

Treatment

The treatments for depression of AD that have been investigated are primarily pharmacological. Nine placebo-controlled trials of antidepressants in dementia (mostly AD) have been completed to date, with mixed results. Selective serotonin reuptake inhibitors (SSRIs), particularly citalopram and sertraline, have been the most commonly tested agents, although two trials used tricyclic antidepressants and one used moclobemide. Four studies demonstrated benefit over placebo, four did not, and one had mixed outcomes. Most of the positive studies limited the mood diagnosis to major depression, whereas most of the negative trials defined depression more broadly.[48] Overall, the methodologies are too disparate to draw firm conclusions, but the most rigorous trial was positive for sertraline on primary depression outcomes and favored the active treatment over placebo for the secondary outcomes of behavioral disturbance, role functioning, and caregiver distress.[60] There is no substantial evidence that antidepressant treatment improves or worsens cognition, regardless of the outcome for depression.[48]

Non-Alzheimer's Dementias

There is a dearth of information on depression in dementias other than AD. Several results suggest that depression may actually be more common in vascular dementia than in AD. Depression in vascular dementia has been associated with abnormal neurological signs such as extrapyramidal symptoms and grasp reflexes, possibly implicating frontal-subcortical circuits.[31] Likewise, depression may be more common in dementia with Lewy bodies than in AD, although results are mixed, with the prevalence reported from 25% to 60%.[61] Some results suggest that apathy may be more common and depression less common in frontotemporal dementia.[62]

AGITATION

Epidemiology

Agitation differs from psychosis and depression of AD in that it may be conceptualized as a single symptom or a symptom complex. The prevalence of agitation in dementia ranges from 20% to 60%, depending on diagnostic definitions used and the population studied.[63] Cohen-Mansfield[64] proposed a formalized definition of agitation as "inappropriate verbal, vocal, or motor activity that is not judged by an outside observer to be an obvious outcome of the needs or confusion of the individual." She also characterized subtypes of agitation that may have important clinical differences, including physical versus verbal and aggressive versus nonaggressive types.[64]

Considerable evidence points to an increase in all types of agitation as the severity of the dementia progresses. Agitation may be quite persistent, as indicated by continued verbal agitation for 3 months in 67% of participants in one sample, despite an average of more than 13 interventions targeting the agitation.[65] Risk factors for agitation are numerous and may differ depending on the subtype of agitation. Verbal agitation appears to be increased by social isolation, sensory impairment, female sex, pain, use of physical restraints, functional impairment, and worse medical status, and possibly by premorbid personality factors.[65] On the other hand, aggression occurs more often in men, in those with more cognitive impairment, and in those with a history of premorbid aggression and conflict with their caregivers.[66] Physically nonaggressive behavior has been linked to worse cognitive status and better physical health.[47]

Evidence for a Distinct Entity

Agitation in dementia often co-occurs with psychosis and depression. There is substantial evidence that verbal agitation is associated with depression, and there may be some relationship to delusions.[47] Psychosis, particularly delusions, and depression occur with increased frequency in aggressive patients and may be a causative factor.[67] Yet, agitation may also be independently linked to several important clinical outcomes, including increased patient mortality, behavioral problems in other residents with dementia in nursing homes, falls, caregiver distress, and early patient institutionalization.[65,68] Agitated behavior among AD patients does not invariably stem from other "primary" psychiatric disturbances, as indicated by the aforementioned cluster/ factor analyses; two of three such studies singled out agitation as distinct from depression, psychosis, and sleep disturbance.[9,10]

Etiology

Because of the variable definitions used for agitation, it is difficult to ascribe it to a single cause. Certain agitated behavior may occur in response to medical illness, physical discomfort, or psychosocial factors. When agitation is severe and persistent in the absence of other clear causes, biological factors intrinsic to dementia may be at play. Several potential biological correlates of agitation in AD have been investigated. Among the abnormalities are changes in frontal and temporal lobe metabolism detected by functional imaging and increased neurofibrillary tangle burden in orbitofrontal and anterior cingulate cortices.[69,70] Neurotransmitter systems have been implicated as well. For example, AD patients with agitation compared with those without agitation had lowered choline acetyltransferase activity in the frontal and temporal lobes and lower choline acetyltransferase/dopamine ratios in the temporal cortex.[71] Serotonergic changes associated with agitation in AD include 1) serotonin transporter gene polymorphisms; 2) altered prolactin levels in a fenfluramine challenge test; 3) altered serotonin$_{1A}$ receptor binding in postmortem samples; and 4) polymorphisms in the serotonin$_{2A}$ receptor.[70,72]

Proposed Criteria

In contrast to psychosis and depression of AD, no expert consensus criteria have been proposed for the diagnosis of agitation in AD. There are several barriers to this occurring. Agitation does not map onto other DSM diagnostic constructs in the way psychosis, depression, and sleep disorder of AD do. Although long recognized as an important and problematic behavior in AD, agitation remains perhaps a more nebulous diagnostic construct. The medical literature on dementia often uses the terms *agitation, behavioral problem,* and *disruptive behavior* interchangeably. Studies of agitation have often included persons with a mixture of dementia diagnoses.

Some may reasonably fear that creating a diagnostic label of agitation may lead to inappropriate use of chemical restraint. Resistance may also stem from the widespread use of the term *agitation* and the consequent reduction in the clinically meaningful information the label conveys. That is to say, there has probably been a clinical tendency to label many behavioral manifestations of dementia as "agitation" without much critical thought or detailed observation to distinguish among various subtypes of behavioral symptoms. Nonetheless, the construct, as defined by Cohen-Mansfield,[64] appears to convey significant clinical information. Using another label for the phenomenon of agitation might help reduce inappropriate "lumping together" of different neuropsychiatric phenomena in dementia. However, this terminology is deeply ingrained in the history of describing behavioral symptoms in dementia. At the least, criteria developed for agitation should make clear the aspects that distinguish this diagnostic label from others and specify that "agitation" should not be indiscriminately applied to all behavioral disturbances. Further study of the subtypes of agitation described by Cohen-Mansfield may provide evidence to guide classification.

Treatment

The first step in the care of the "agitated" patient is a complete assessment to evaluate for proximal causes of the agitation. Such causes may include pain or untreated medical illness, in which case masking the "agitated" behavior with sedating agents would have potentially harmful consequences. Agitation co-occurring with depression, psychosis, or insomnia may respond to treatments targeting these syndromes. Anecdotal experience suggests that pharmacological management of agitated behaviors that do not have an identifiable medical cause and do not occur in the context of a more readily treatable behavioral syndrome is often disappointing in its effectiveness.

Although it may be a more difficult construct to define, idiopathic agitation has attracted many treatment trials in dementia patients. The most commonly used first-generation antipsychotic, haloperidol, was found in a meta-analysis to be beneficial for dementia patients with aggression but not for agitation more generally.[73] Randomized controlled studies with risperidone and olanzapine show modest efficacy for reducing aggression and overall agitation in AD.[74] The evidence for the efficacy of other agents in improving agitation in dementia is scarce. Mood stabilizers have been used to reduce impulsivity and aggression in other clinical populations, prompting exploration of their use in agitation in dementia, but the results are inconclusive. Limited data show some efficacy of the SSRI citalopram, although trials with other SSRIs have been negative.[75] A systematic review of psychosocial treatments for agitation in dementia found 19 randomized controlled trials, with only 8 of these being judged as "high quality." This review indicated that there is some evidence for the use of psychomotor group therapy to reduce aggression in institutionalized AD patients.[64]

Non-Alzheimer's Dementias

Agitation occurs across all diagnostic categories of dementia. The studies that have directly compared these symptoms in different forms of dementia have thus far largely failed to indicate any significant differences in the prevalence among the various dementias. A few studies have shown differences, such as one finding agitation more frequently among patients with frontotemporal dementia (91%) than among patients with AD (68%).[32] Another study found less "activity disturbance" in dementia with Lewy bodies than in AD, but motor symptoms and gait impairment could account for this finding.[62]

SLEEP DISTURBANCE IN ALZHEIMER'S DISEASE

Although often symptomatic of other medical and/or psychiatric comorbidity, sleep disturbances may occur as a primary symptom in AD. Sleep problems occur in 19%–44% of clinic and community samples of patients with AD.[76] Sleep disturbances have been independently associated with caregiver distress, patient institutionalization, and increased cognitive and functional impairments in patients.[76] The characteristic changes that occur in sleep architecture in AD appear in some respects to be an exaggeration of the changes that occur in healthy older adults but also include more distinctive changes, such as a decrease in the percentage of sleep time spent in rapid eye movement sleep.[15] Potential biological explanations for disturbed sleep in AD include deterioration of the cholinergic system, brainstem regions that regulate sleep, and the suprachiasmatic nucleus of the thalamus, which regulates circadian rhythms.[15,77]

Environmental factors that may affect sleep in AD include decreased daylight exposure, decreased daytime activity levels, increased time spent awake in bed, and increased exposure to nighttime noises in institutional settings.[78] Primary sleep disorders, such as restless legs syndrome and obstructive sleep apnea, become more prevalent with age and may complicate the diagnostic picture of sleep problems in dementia.[15]

Sleep disturbance in AD attracted a third consensus group to develop proposed diagnostic criteria for this clinical syndrome.[15] The criteria include symptoms of insomnia, hypersomnia, and circadian rhythm disturbances, although these are not included as specifiers. Exclusionary criteria include other obvious medical, psychiatric, substance-related, or primary sleep disorder causes of the symptoms. Validation of these criteria remains to be demonstrated in a systematic fashion. Treatment studies for sleep disorders in dementia are sparse. The largest and best-designed pharmacological study for sleep disturbance in AD thus far found no benefit for patients using melatonin versus those receiving placebo.[15] A recent review of light therapy in dementia concluded that among the six randomized controlled trials thus far, the results hold promise but are inconclusive regarding the effects on sleep–wake parameters.[79] A randomized controlled trial was positive for a psychosocial intervention with AD patients that combined attention to improved sleep hygiene, regular daily exercise, and increased daytime light exposure.[80]

Future Research Directions

Major advances in understanding neuropsychiatric symptoms in dementia have been made since DSM was last revised. However, much remains to be learned in order to maximize meaningful and evidence-based changes in these diagnoses for DSM-V (see Table 6–1).[81] The existence of provisional criteria with good face va-

---

TABLE 6–1.   Future research needs

Validate proposed diagnostic categories and subcategories

Repeat epidemiological studies using validated diagnostic criteria

Identify how best to conceptualize syndrome overlap, heterogeneity, and comorbidity

Refine outcome measures for clinical trials (symptom scales developed for and validated in this population measures of quality of life, functional ability, caregiver health, and economic outcomes)

Identify at-risk populations (e.g., patients with mild cognitive impairment) for longitudinal study

Apply biotechnologies (e.g., functional neuroimaging and genetics/genomics) to identify syndrome etiologies, subtypes, risk factors, and treatment mediators/moderators

Expand study into non-Alzheimer's dementias

Identify potential prevention strategies for at-risk patients

Identify novel pharmacological targets specific to syndromes (e.g., corticotropin-releasing factor for depression) or specific to dementia etiology (e.g., β-amyloid for Alzheimer's disease)

---

lidity for three neuropsychiatric syndromes in AD serves as a starting point. Efforts to validate these criteria in diverse samples of AD patients will yield important information in upcoming years. Once valid criteria are available, existing epidemiological research should be replicated using these new criteria.

Despite best efforts at categorizing these psychiatric symptoms in dementia, some problems may remain unresolved in the near future. Examples include heterogeneity within any diagnostic grouping and comorbidity of diagnoses attributable to co-occurrence of separate phenomena or diagnostic overlap. Ascertaining whether polysymptomatic cases represent subtypes within a prevailing symptom category, co-occurrence of two disorders, or a separate diagnosis distinct from the two individual diagnoses will require considerable systematic study. More definitive answers are likely to come from better understanding of the neurobiological changes that underlie these symptoms.

Fortunately, this is a time of significant advancement in the technological tools used to understand the biology underlying complex psychiatric phenomena. Functional neuroimaging and genetic/genomic studies have substantial promise and have already been applied to the study of neuropsychiatric syndromes in dementia. Functional neuroimaging and genetic analysis may help to identify mediators and moderators of treatment response or nonresponse.

The bulk of knowledge about neuropsychiatric syndromes pertains to AD specifically or to dementia more broadly. Yet the increasing recognition of vascular dementia and dementia with Lewy bodies dictates a need for similar research in these disorders. Some neuropsychiatric diagnoses developed for AD may map well onto other dementias, but important differences may exist in the prognosis and treatment response of neuropsychiatric syndromes according to the type of dementia. While looking for important biological factors, researchers should simultaneously explore further how sociocultural variables may differentially affect psychiatric symptoms in patients with the same underlying biological pathology. Culture may have a profound influence on idioms of distress and societal interpretations of symptoms, and this may produce different illness phenotypes from identical biological pathology. The need for cross-cultural validation also applies to rating scales used to assess the severity and treatment response of neuropsychiatric syndromes.

One unique aspect of studying dementia (compared with other neuropsychiatric illnesses) is the emerging evidence for a reasonably reliable and valid prodrome (mild cognitive impairment) that portends the development of dementia, particularly the Alzheimer's type, in a large portion of cases. This population offers a unique opportunity to characterize biological and psychosocial factors associated with the transition from a premorbid phase to the onset of specific neuropsychiatric syndromes. Studying at-risk populations may also assist the development of preventive interventions.

Refining diagnostic classification will improve treatment trials as well. Identifying a homogeneous target population could improve the power to detect the positive effects of treatments that otherwise appear ineffective because their therapeutic effects are diluted by inclusion of participants inappropriate for the trial. In addition, incorporation of other, more meaningful outcome measures (including functional, quality-of-life, caregiver-oriented, and economic measures) will be crucial for evaluating treatments. However, methodological improvements alone are unlikely to be enough. Currently available psychotropic medications were developed for syndromes in younger adults, and enthusiasm for their use in dementia is lukewarm based on results from current trials. Ultimately, most pharmacological and psychosocial treatments developed thus far in psychiatry have not been designed with the degenerating brain of dementia patients in mind. Treatments for neuropsychiatric syndromes in dementia face the obstacle of having to act in a milieu that is by definition losing the very substrate on which these treatments act. Many investigators are using specific molecular targets, such as β-amyloid and tau protein in AD, to develop new therapies. As new agents, such as β- and γ-secretase inhibitors, reach the point of clinical trials, it will be important to identify their potential therapeutic effects on neuropsychiatric syndromes in AD, in addition to the cognitive and functional measures that are likely to be the primary outcomes examined initially.

The diagnostic classification of all psychiatric illnesses remains suboptimal, and it is unlikely that neuropsychiatric diagnoses developed for dementia in DSM-V will represent a destination; rather, they will represent another step in the journey toward diagnostic clarity. Nevertheless, the neuropsychiatric syndromes of AD have undergone considerable study and refinement, and research in the near future can help develop diagnostic criteria with improved reliability and validity. These syndromes are so pervasive and intrinsic to dementia, and so catastrophic for patients and caregivers alike, that we must endeavor to categorize them more coherently in the hopes of facilitating their detection and appropriate treatment.

References

1. Assal F, Cummings JL: Neuropsychiatric symptoms in the dementias. Curr Opin Neurol 15:445–450, 2002.
2. Murman DL, Colenda CC: The economic impact of neuropsychiatric symptoms in Alzheimer's disease: can drugs ease the burden? Pharmacoeconomics 23:227–242, 2005.
3. American Psychiatric Association: Diagnostic and Statistical Manual of Mental Disorders, 3rd Edition. Washington, DC, American Psychiatric Association, 1980.
4. American Psychiatric Association: Diagnostic and Statistical Manual of Mental Disorders, 3rd Edition, Revised. Washington, DC, American Psychiatric Association, 1987.
5. American Psychiatric Association: Diagnostic and Statistical Manual of Mental Disorders, 4th Edition. Washington, DC, American Psychiatric Association, 1994.
6. American Psychiatric Association: Diagnostic and Statistical Manual of Mental Disorders, 4th Edition, Text Revision. Washington, DC, American Psychiatric Association, 2000.
7. Eastham JH, Jeste DV: Differentiating behavioral disturbances of dementia from drug side effects. Int Psychogeriatr 8:429–434, 1996.
8. Lyketsos CG, Breitner JC, Rabins PV: An evidence-based proposal for the classification of neuropsychiatric disturbance in Alzheimer's disease. Int J Geriatr Psychiatry 16:1037–1042, 2001.
9. Schreinzer D, Ballaban T, Brannath W, et al: Components of behavioral pathology in dementia. Int J Geriatr Psychiatry 20:137–145, 2005.
10. Harwood DG, Ownby RL, Barker WW, et al. The Behavioral Pathology in Alzheimer's Disease Scale (BEHAVE-AD): factor structure among community-dwelling Alzheimer's disease patients. Int J Geriatr Psychiatry 13:793–800, 1998.
11. Zubenko GS, Rosen J, Sweet RA, et al: Impact of psychiatric hospitalization on behavioral complications of Alzheimer's disease. Am J Psychiatry 149:1484–1491, 1992.
12. Lyketsos CG, Sheppard JE, Steinberg M, et al: Neuropsychiatric disturbance in Alzheimer's disease clusters into three groups: the Cache County Study. Int J Geriatr Psychiatry 16:1043–1053, 1992.
13. Jeste DV, Finkel SI: Psychosis of Alzheimer's disease and related dementias: diagnostic criteria for a distinct syndrome. Am J Geriatr Psychiatry 8:29–34, 2000.

14. Olin JT, Katz IR, Meyers BS, et al: Provisional diagnostic criteria for depression of Alzheimer disease: rationale and background. Am J Geriatr Psychiatry 10:129–141, 2002.

15. Yesavage JA, Friedman L, Ancoli-Israel S, et al: Development of diagnostic criteria for defining sleep disturbance in Alzheimer's disease. J Geriatr Psychiatry Neurol 16:131–139, 2003.

16. Ropacki SA, Jeste DV: Epidemiology of and risk factors for psychosis of Alzheimer's disease: a review of 55 studies published from 1990 to 2003. Am J Psychiatry 162:2022–2030, 2005.

17. Paulsen JS, Salmon DP, Thal LJ, et al: Incidence of and risk factors for hallucinations and delusions in patients with probable AD. Neurology 54:1965–1971, 2000.

18. Jeste DV, Wragg RE, Salmon DP, et al: Cognitive deficits of patients with Alzheimer's disease with and without delusions. Am J Psychiatry 149:184–189, 1992.

19. Zubenko GS, Moossy J, Martinez AJ, et al: Neuropathologic and neurochemical correlates of psychosis in primary dementia. Arch Neurol 48:619–624, 1991.

20. Forstl H, Dalgalarrondo P, Riecher-Rossler A, et al: Organic factors and the clinical features of late paranoid psychosis: a comparison with Alzheimer's disease and normal aging. Acta Psychiatr Scand 89:335–340, 1994.

21. Rosen J, Zubenko GS: Emergence of psychosis and depression in the longitudinal evaluation of Alzheimer's disease. Biol Psychiatry 29:224–232, 1991.

22. Sweet RA, Nimgaonkar VL, Devlin B, et al: Psychotic symptoms in Alzheimer disease: evidence for a distinct phenotype. Mol Psychiatry 8:383–392, 2003.

23. Lopez OL, Brenner RP, Becker JT, et al: EEG spectral abnormalities and psychosis as predictors of cognitive and functional decline in probable Alzheimer's disease. Neurology 48:1521–1525, 1997.

24. Kotrla KJ, Chacko RC, Harper RG, et al: SPECT findings on psychosis in Alzheimer's disease. Am J Psychiatry 152:1470–1475, 1995.

25. Geroldi C, Bresciani L, Zanetti O, et al: Regional brain atrophy in patients with mild Alzheimer's disease and delusions. Int Psychogeriatr 14:365–378, 2002.

26. Hoeh N, Gyulai L, Weintraub D, et al: Pharmacologic management of psychosis in the elderly: a critical review. J Geriatr Psychiatry Neurol 16:213–218, 2003.

27. Jeste DV, Okamoto A, Napolitano J, et al: Low incidence of persistent tardive dyskinesia in elderly patients with dementia treated with risperidone. Am J Psychiatry. 157:1150–1155, 2000.

28. Hammerstrom K: Atypical antipsychotic drugs, dementia, and risk of death (letter). JAMA 295:496, 2006.

29. Schneider LS, Tariot PN, Lyketsos CG, et al: National Institute of Mental Health—Clinical Antipsychotic Trials of Intervention Effectiveness (CATIE): Alzheimer disease trial methodology. Am J Geriatr Psychiatry 9:346–360, 2001.

30. Del Ser T, McKeith I, Anand R, et al: Dementia with Lewy bodies: findings from an international multicentre study. Int J Geriatr Psychiatry 15:1034–1045, 2000.

31. O'Brien J: Behavioral symptoms in vascular cognitive impairment and vascular dementia. Int Psychogeriatr 15:133–138, 2003.

32. Srikanth S, Nagaraja AV, Ratnavalli E: Neuropsychiatric symptoms in dementia—frequency, relationship to dementia severity and comparison in Alzheimer's disease, vascular dementia and frontotemporal dementia. J Neurol Sci 236:43–48, 2005.

33. Zubenko GS: Major depressive disorder in Alzheimer's disease, in Late Life Depression. Edited by Roose S, Sackheim H. New York, Oxford University Press, 2004, pp 361–369.

34. Merriam AE, Aronson MK, Gaston P, et al: The psychiatric symptoms of Alzheimer's disease. J Am Geriatr Soc 36:7–12, 1988.

35. Lee HB, Lyketsos CG: Depression in Alzheimer's disease: heterogeneity and related issues. Biol Psychiatry 54:353–362, 2003.

36. Zubenko GS, Zubenko WN, McPherson S, et al: A collaborative study of the emergence and clinical features of the major depressive syndrome of Alzheimer's disease. Am J Psychiatry 160:857–866, 2003.

37. Wilson RS, Barnes LL, Mendes de Leon CF, et al: Depressive symptoms, cognitive decline, and risk of AD in older persons. Neurology 59:364–370, 2002.

38. Zubenko GS, Zubenko WN, Spiker DG, et al: Malignancy of recurrent, early-onset major depression: a family study. Am J Med Genet 105:690–699, 2001.

39. Weissman MM, Leaf PJ, Tischler GL, et al: Affective disorders in five United States communities. Psychol Med 18:141–153, 1988.

40. Rifai AH, Mulsant BH, Sweet RA, et al: A study of elderly suicide attempters admitted to an inpatient psychiatric unit. Am J Geriatr Psychiatry 1:126–135, 1993.

41. Pearlson GD, Ross CA, Lohr WD, et al: Association between family history of affective disorder and the depressive syndrome of Alzheimer's disease. Am J Psychiatry 147: 452–456, 1990.

42. Fahim S, van Duijn CM, Baker FM, et al: A study of familial aggregation of depression, dementia and Parkinson's disease. Eur J Epidemiol 14:233–238, 1998.

43. Heun R, Papassotiropoulos A, Jessen F, et al: A family study of Alzheimer's disease and early and late-onset depression in elderly patients. Arch Gen Psychiatry 58:190–196, 2001.

44. Starkstein SE, Petracca G, Chemerinski E, et al: Syndromic validity of apathy in Alzheimer's disease. Am J Psychiatry 158:872–877, 2001.

45. Holthoff VA, Beuthien-Baumann B, Kalbe E, et al: Regional cerebral metabolism in early Alzheimer's disease with clinically significant apathy or depression. Biol Psychiatry 57:412–421, 2005.

46. Bassiony MM, Warren A, Rosenblatt A, et al: The relationship between delusions and depression in Alzheimer's disease. Int J Geriatr Psychiatry 17:549–556, 2002.

47. Cohen-Mansfield L, Werner P: Longitudinal predictors of nonaggressive agitated behaviors in the elderly. Int J Geriatr Psychiatry 14:831–844, 1999.

48. Lyketsos CG, Olin J: Depression in Alzheimer's disease: overview and treatment. Biol Psychiatry 52:243–252, 2002.

49. Zubenko GS, Moossy J: Major depression in primary dementia: clinical and neuropathological correlates. Arch Neurol 45:1182–1186, 1988.

50. Zweig RM, Ross CA, Hedreen JC, et al: The neuropathology of aminergic nuclei in Alzheimer's disease. Ann Neurol 24:233–242, 1988.

51. Chan-Palay V: Depression and senile dementia of the Alzheimer type: catecholamine changes in the locus coeruleus—basis for therapy. Dementia 1:253–261, 1990.

52. Forstl H, Burns A, Luthert P, et al: Clinical and neuropathological correlates of depression in Alzheimer's disease. Psychol Med 22:877–884, 1992.

53. Zubenko GS, Moossy J, Kopp U: Neurochemical correlates of major depression in primary dementia. Arch Neurol 47:209–214, 1990.
54. Zubenko GS: Clinicopathologic and neurochemical correlates of major depression and psychosis in primary dementia. Int Psychogeriatr 8 (suppl 3):219–223, 1996.
55. Krishnan KRR, Tupler LA, Ritchie JC, et al: Apolipoprotein E-4 frequency in geriatric depression. Biol Psychiatry 40:69–71, 1996.
56. Scarmeas N, Brandt J, Albert M, et al: Association between the APOE genotype and psychopathologic symptoms in Alzheimer's disease. Neurology 58:1182–1188, 2002.
57. Hirono N, Mori E, Ishii K, et al: Frontal lobe hypometabolism and depression in Alzheimer's disease. Neurology 50:380–383, 1998.
58. Hirono N, Mori E, Ishii K, et al: Alteration of regional cerebral glucose utilization with delusions in Alzheimer's disease. J Neuropsychiatry Clin Neurosci 10:433–439, 1998.
59. Starkstein SE, Jorge R, Mizrahi R, et al: The construct of minor and major depression in Alzheimer's disease. Am J Psychiatry 162:2086–2093, 2005.
60. Lyketsos CG, Del Campo L, Steinberg M, et al: Treating depression in Alzheimer disease: efficacy and safety of sertraline therapy, and the benefits of depression reduction: the DIADS. Arch Gen Psychiatry 60:737–746, 2003.
61. Samuels SC, Brickman AM, Burd JA, et al: Depression in autopsy-confirmed dementia with Lewy bodies and Alzheimer's disease. Mt Sinai J Med 71:55–62, 2004.
62. Engelborghs S, Maertens K, Nagels G, et al: Neuropsychiatric symptoms of dementia: cross-sectional analysis from a prospective, longitudinal Belgian study. Int J Geriatr Psychiatry 20:1028–1037, 2005.
63. Aalten P, de Vugt ME, Lousberg R, et al: Behavioral problems in dementia: a factor analysis of the neuropsychiatric inventory. Dement Geriatr Cogn Disord 15:99–105, 2003.
64. Cohen-Mansfield J: Nonpharmacologic interventions for inappropriate behaviors in dementia: a review and critique. Am J Geriatr Psychiatry 9:361–381, 2001.
65. McMinn B, Draper B: Vocally disruptive behaviour in dementia: development of an evidence based practice guideline. Aging Ment Health 9:16–24, 2005.
66. Hamel M, Gold DP, Andres D, et al: Predictors and consequences of aggressive behavior by community-based dementia patients. Gerontologist 30:206–211, 1990.
67. Deutsch LH, Bylsma FW, Rovner BW, et al: Psychosis and physical aggression in probable Alzheimer's disease. Am J Psychiatry 148:1159–1163, 1991.
68. Allen RS, Burgio LD, Fisher SE, et al: Behavioral characteristics of agitated nursing home residents with dementia at the end of life. Gerontologist 45:661–666, 2005.
69. Sultzer DL, Mahler ME, Mandelkern MA, et al: The relationship between psychiatric symptoms and regional cortical metabolism in Alzheimer's disease. J Neuropsychiatry Clin Neurosci 7:476–484, 1995.
70. Tekin S, Mega MS, Masterman DM, et al: Orbitofrontal and anterior cingulate cortex neurofibrillary tangle burden is associated with agitation in Alzheimer disease. Ann Neurol 49:355–361, 2001.
71. Trinh NH, Hoblyn J, Mohanty S, et al: Efficacy of cholinesterase inhibitors in the treatment of neuropsychiatric symptoms and functional impairment in Alzheimer disease: a meta-analysis. JAMA 289:210–216, 2003.
72. Zarros A, Kalopita KS, Tsakiris ST: Serotoninergic impairment and aggressive behavior in Alzheimer's disease. Acta Neurobiol Exp (Wars) 65:277–286, 2005.

73. Lonergan E, Luxenberg J, Colford J: Haloperidol for agitation in dementia. Cochrane Database Syst Rev. 4:CD002852, 2001.

74. Ballard C, Waite J: The effectiveness of atypical antipsychotics for the treatment of aggression and psychosis in Alzheimer's disease. Cochrane Database Syst Rev 1:CD003476, 2006.

75. Bharani N, Snowden M: Evidence-based interventions for nursing home residents with dementia-related behavioral symptoms. Psychiatr Clin North Am 28:985–1005, 2005.

76. McCurry SM, Reynolds CF, Ancoli-Israel S, et al: Treatment of sleep disturbance in Alzheimer's disease. Sleep Med Rev 4:603–628, 2000.

77. Petit D, Gagnon JF, Fantini ML, et al: Sleep and quantitative EEG in neurodegenerative disorders. J Psychosom Res 56:487–496, 2004.

78. Ancoli-Israel S, Gehrman P, Martin JL, et al: Increased light exposure consolidates sleep and strengthens circadian rhythms in severe Alzheimer's disease patients. Behav Sleep Med 1:22–36, 2003.

79. Skjerve A, Bjorvatn B, Holsten F: Light therapy for behavioural and psychological symptoms of dementia. Int J Geriatr Psychiatry 19:516–522, 2004.

80. McCurry SM, Gibbons LE, Logsdon RG, et al: Nighttime insomnia treatment and education for Alzheimer's disease: a randomized, controlled trial. J Am Geriatr Soc 53:793–802, 2005.

81. Jeste DV, Blazer DG, First M: Aging-related diagnostic variations: need for diagnostic criteria appropriate for elderly psychiatric patients. Biol Psychiatry 58:265–271, 2005.

7

BIOMARKERS IN THE DIAGNOSIS OF ALZHEIMER'S DISEASE

Are We Ready?

Trey Sunderland, M.D.
Harald Hampel, M.D.
Masatoshi Takeda, M.D., Ph.D.
Karen T. Putnam, M.S.
Robert M. Cohen, M.D., Ph.D.

The potential usefulness of biomarkers in Alzheimer's disease (AD) is generally accepted, at least on a theoretical basis within the research community. Clinically, there is a long history of using biomarkers as diagnostic measures or surrogate markers for therapeutic interventions and prognosis in general medicine,[1,2] but there are no such markers in geriatric neuropsychiatry.[3] The underlying pathophysiology

This work was supported by a grant from the National Institute of Mental Health (Z01 MH00330-14).

This chapter is reprinted from Sunderland T, Hampel H, Takeda M, et al.: "Biomarkers in the Diagnosis of Alzheimer's Disease: Are We Ready?" *Journal of Geriatric Psychiatry and Neurology* 19:172–179, 2006. Used with permission.

of a neurodegenerative illness such as AD makes it a prime candidate for such discovery. Nonetheless, the field has been relatively slow to move in this direction. Furthermore, there are many misunderstandings about the use of biomarkers in AD research. Some of these misunderstandings revolve around the confusion over whether biomarkers are meant for diagnostic purposes or to help monitor therapeutic effects in clinical trials. In this review, we primarily address the potential usefulness of biomarkers in the diagnosis and management of AD and the future challenges to incorporating this approach more formally into our diagnostic criteria.

For more than a century, AD has been diagnosed based on clinical criteria antemortem and confirmed by pathological criteria at autopsy.[4,5] Although multiple sets of national and international criteria are in wide use,[6-8] they all share the basic characteristic that AD is diagnosed by virtue of clinically significant cognitive changes over time in the absence of other known causes of dementia (Table 7–1). Given that postmortem studies report agreements of approximately 85% between the clinical criteria and the pathological confirmations,[4,5,9,10] one might even question why one needs to improve on these criteria and how biomarkers might help in this process. Here lies the first of many important misconceptions about the AD clinical diagnosis. It is very unlikely that the clinical accuracy of an AD diagnosis is anywhere close to 85%–90% at the time of most initial clinical diagnoses. There are just too many uncertainties and clinical vagaries that make a definitive diagnosis impossible at the early stages of the illness, especially as the general awareness of AD increases and patients come to the clinic earlier and earlier in their course of illness. Rather, the diagnosis probably only approaches this high level of accuracy as the clinician follows the individual patient over many years or compares multiple assessment instruments,[11] thereby gradually eliminating other potential confounds.

Postmortem studies are, by their very nature, retrospective studies that generally use only the most recent clinical diagnosis, which integrates years of observations, not just the initial diagnostic impression at the earliest stage of the illness. Concordance between the first-impression clinical diagnoses and the final pathological observations would most likely be much lower, perhaps only 50%.[12] Given the initial clinical confusion between AD and other diagnoses such as depression, frontotemporal dementia, Lewy body dementia, Parkinson's dementia, and the many other neurodegenerative illnesses in the differential diagnosis, there are undoubtedly many opportunities for improved diagnostic accuracy, especially at the earliest stages of evaluation. Specific, pathophysiologically linked biomarkers are therefore particularly interesting targets in this early diagnostic process.

Over the past 5–10 years, multiple candidates have emerged in the literature as potential diagnostic biomarkers for AD. These purported biomarkers have ranged from an ophthalmologic sensitivity test to genetic markers to cerebrospinal fluid

TABLE 7–1. Diagnostic criteria for Alzheimer's disease according to ICD-10,[7] DSM-IV-TR,[8] and NINCDS-ADRDA[6]

	ICD-10	DSM-IV-TR	NINCDS-ADRDA
Onset age	Early (below age 65) and late (age 65 or more)	Early (age 65 and below) and late (after age 65)	Between ages 40 and 90, most often after age 65
Disease course	Gradual onset and continuing cognitive decline. Plateaus in the course of the disease possible	Gradual onset and continuing cognitive decline	Progressive deterioration of memory and other cognitive functions
Duration	Presence of symptoms for at least 6 months	No requirement	No requirement
Cognitive profile	Decline in memory and decline in other cognitive abilities, representing a deterioration from a previously higher level of performance	Multiple cognitive deficits including memory and at least one of the following: aphasia, apraxia, agnosia, disturbance in executive functions	Dementia syndrome with deficits in 2 or more cognitive domains; progressive worsening of memory and other cognitive functions
Impairments in activities of daily living	Impairment in personal activities of daily living such as washing, dressing, eating, personal hygiene, use of toilet	Impairment in occupational or social functioning attributable to cognitive deficits, representing a decline from a previously higher level of functioning	Not explicitly required for the diagnosis, should be assessed, supports a diagnosis of probable AD
Consciousness	Absence of clouding of consciousness	Deficits do not occur except during the course of a delirium	No disturbance of consciousness

TABLE 7–1. Diagnostic criteria for Alzheimer's disease according to ICD-10,[7] DSM-IV-TR,[8] and NINCDS-ADRDA[6] *(continued)*

	ICD-10	DSM-IV-TR	NINCDS-ADRDA
Exclusion criteria	No evidence from history, physical examination, or special investigations for any other possible cause of dementia or alcohol or drug abuse	Exclusion of other CNS conditions causing progressive deficits in memory and cognition, systemic conditions causing dementia, substance-induced conditions, and other Axis I disorders	Sudden, apoplectic onset; focal neurologic findings; seizures or gait disorders at the onset or very early in the course of the illness

Note.   AD=Alzheimer's disease; CNS=central nervous system; DSM-IV-TR=*Diagnostic and Statistical Manual of Mental Disorders*, 4th Edition, Text Revision; ICD=*International Classification of Disease*; NINCDS-ADRDA=National Institute of Neurological and Communicative Disorders and Stroke–Alzheimer's Disease and Related Disorders Association.

TABLE 7–2. Selected examples of proposed biomarkers in the diagnosis of Alzheimer's disease

Category	Selected markers	References
Blood markers	C1q, IL-6RC, oxysterols, homocysteine, APOE levels, isoprostane, α-1-antichymotrypsin, 3-nitrotyrosine	19, 48–54
Brain imaging	CT, MRI, SPECT, PET, ^{1}H-MRS, fMRI, PET ligands	16, 55–60
Cerebrospinal fluid	β-amyloid$_{1-42}$, β-amyloid$_{1-40}$, total tau and p-tau	21, 28–30, 61–66

Note. APOE=apolipoprotein E; CT=computed tomography; fMRI=functional MRI; IL=interleukin; MRI=magnetic resonance imaging; ^{1}H-MRS=^{1}H-labeled magnetic resonance spectroscopy; PET=positron emission tomography; p-tau = hyperphosphorylated tau; SPECT=single photon emission computed tomography.

(CSF) peptide measures of amyloid and tau to urinary measures of brain peptides and a multitude of neuroimaging parameters, and the list continues to grow steadily (Table 7–2).[13–22] Some potential diagnostic measures have entered the scientific literature or even the commercial marketplace with much fanfare, only to be abandoned later because of a lack of replication or reliability across research centers (i.e., tropicamide, urinary neural thread protein). Because we are focusing on the near-term usefulness of biomarkers in the diagnosis and evaluation of AD, it is beyond the scope of this chapter to exhaustively review the history and science behind each individual biomarker. Rather, we will concentrate on those biomarkers with the most convincing track record of scientific replication and biological relatedness to AD.

Given the central importance of β-amyloid plaques and neurofibrillary tangles in the neuropathological diagnosis of AD at autopsy,[4,5] it is a reasonable assumption that the underlying components of these pathognomonic features might be good targets as clinical biomarkers of AD. In fact, studies of antemortem biomarkers have focused on the β-amyloid and tau components from several human tissues, including brain biopsy material, CSF, and peripheral blood.[21,23–25] Specifically, CSF β-amyloid$_{1-42}$, β-amyloid$_{1-40}$, total tau, and hyperphosphorylated tau (p-tau) have emerged as the major biomarkers of interest.[14,17,18,21,26] Although other biomarkers may eventually emerge as wonderful candidates for future research, these CSF markers are currently best poised to make a difference in the early diagnosis of AD.

In defining an ideal diagnostic biomarker, the National Institute on Aging Working Group outlined several key factors, including fundamental relatedness to the illness, validation, specificity, and reliability. Furthermore, this group suggested that the ideal biomarkers should be noninvasive, simple to perform, and inexpensive.[27] Thus far, the most convincing data in the published literature come from CSF studies suggesting a decrease in β-amyloid and an increase in tau when comparing AD with control participants.[21,28–30] There is even a commercial assay available for this combination of tests that reports 90% sensitivity and 80% specificity for the diagnosis of AD (Athena Diagnostics, Worcester, MA). Yet this commercial test is performed only a few hundred times per month throughout the United States (Athena Diagnostics, personal communication).

If the diagnostic sensitivity and specificity of a commercially available test for AD are so good, why is this test not used more frequently? Perhaps clinicians have ignored the impressive specificity and sensitivity numbers of this CSF biomarker test because of the perceived difficulties associated with obtaining the required lumbar puncture. Perhaps the clinicians believe there is no diagnostic advantage to the additional procedure compared with noninvasive cognitive testing. Perhaps it is the cost of the assay (as of July 2006, Athena charged $1,075 for a battery of CSF biomarkers, including β-amyloid$_{1-42}$, total tau, and p-tau). All of these issues may contribute to the general underutilization of the assay, but most likely, it is the lack of specific and significant disease-altering treatment options that causes clinicians to hesitate. If better, more pathophysiologically relevant therapies were introduced, and if the therapies were linked with a more specific diagnosis of AD, this hesitancy to use biomarkers of all kinds might change dramatically.

Given that the extant literature on biomarkers is already extensive, especially with respect to the CSF peptide biomarkers, one might ask what more needs to be accomplished scientifically before this biomarker approach is better accepted in the diagnostic nomenclature. For the purposes of this discussion, we focus our comments on three specific but overlapping issues, because the scientific thresholds for answering each question may be quite different.

1. Biomarkers in the diagnosis of AD
2. Biomarkers to monitor therapy in AD
3. Biomarkers as a prognostic measure of AD risk

The amount of published information varies tremendously for each of these topics. Because progress is being made steadily, the diagnostic nomenclature may soon need to reflect these advances.

Biomarkers in the Diagnosis of Alzheimer's Disease

As noted earlier, the diagnostic sensitivity and specificity in differentiating AD from control populations in research studies are already quite good (85%–90%), at least with the most advanced of the currently available CSF biomarkers.[17,21,22,31] This dichotomous differentiation should alone provide a strong rationale for the immediate introduction of biomarker assays into future *Diagnostic and Statistical Manual of Mental Disorders* (DSM) diagnostic criteria, especially because this diagnostic accuracy is available at early stages of the clinical syndrome, long before autopsy verification. However, there are very few markers beyond the CSF peptides for which sufficient data exist across multiple centers to build such a claim. Furthermore, the testing of sensitivity and specificity measures becomes more difficult when multiple diagnostic entities are included in the differential comparisons, as would, of course, be the case in any realistic clinical setting, and the very lack of autopsy confirmation does introduce a certain circularity to the diagnostic labeling process. Although some differential diagnostic data are already published,[32] the sensitivity and specificity are much less definitive, even for the CSF peptides with the longest track record.

We have already addressed some of the reasons these CSF tests might be underused (i.e., expense, general difficulty obtaining a lumbar puncture, perceived lack of advantage over the purely clinical differentiation, a lack of compelling therapeutic options for earlier or more definitive diagnosis), but still, clear improvements can be made to the tests to increase the value of these biomarkers when better potential therapeutic options are available. For instance, there is currently a lack of consensus in the research community as to which single biomarker or group of biomarkers is the best indicator of AD. Even within the most developed but narrow field of CSF biomarkers, there is some controversy as to whether CSF β-amyloid or tau is a better potential diagnostic measure. Using both measures in a nomogram is an attractive solution to this problem, but there still is the question of whether p-tau is more accurate than total tau, and, if so, whether one should measure p-tau$_{181}$, p-tau$_{191}$ or p-tau$_{231}$.[33]

Developing a prospective CSF bank with representative samples obtained from individuals throughout the course of AD might be one approach to solving this problem. Then, comparing the pattern of CSF changes with the pathology of AD at autopsy would provide a powerful scientific study of the relationship between CSF peptides, diagnosis, and progression of pathology. However, this type of longitudinal project is difficult in scope and expense. Another more practical and economical approach might include the cross-sectional comparisons of CSF peptides at different stages of AD versus controls, perhaps with a more modest longitudinal perspective included. An even more direct clinicopathological research project would be to compare CSF and brain peptides at different stages of AD versus controls, using brain biopsy specimens as the gold standard for neuropathological evidence of AD. Although brain biopsy may seem unnecessarily invasive and impractical at this point, the relative risk–benefit ratio of this research approach would change dramatically if potentially toxic AD therapies or preventive regimens eventually become available. A less invasive but theoretically similar approach might include the combination of CSF biomarkers with brain imaging, especially imaging using potentially pathophysiologically relevant neuroimaging ligands such as Pittsburgh Compound B (PIB).[34]

From a simply practical perspective, laboratory techniques in the measurement of CSF peptides (or the development and use of specific neuroimaging tracers) must be more consistent and reliable across laboratories. Although the relative ratios of specific CSF peptides in AD versus control populations are fairly consistent in the published literature, there is currently far too much variance in the actual quantification of these individual biomarkers when compared across research centers.[21] The choice of antibodies, specific assay techniques, and other sources of variance must be closely examined to make the assays more consistent and readily applicable to a general clinical situation. Likewise, the lumbar puncture procedure itself can be streamlined and improved to markedly reduce the threat of lumbar puncture headaches,[35,36] thereby minimizing one of the major clinical impediments to its use in a routine diagnostic evaluation.

Biomarkers to Monitor Therapy in Alzheimer's Disease

Although we have thus far focused mostly on the use of biomarkers in the diagnostic evaluation of AD, there are other potential uses of biomarkers in the clinical monitoring of AD. For instance, the quantitative pattern of biomarkers may change predictably during the course of AD. Currently, most clinicians and researchers alike think of AD in relatively simplistic clinical stages (i.e., mild, moderate, and severe), and for many years, the diagnostic distinctions between these stages have been based primarily on cognitive variables and activities of daily living.[37]

Biomarkers offer the opportunity to gather a quantitative parameter of change over the course of AD. Of course, it is possible that the biomarkers will follow the clinical pattern and add little to the description of the illness. But it is also possible that there will be distinct biological stages of the illness that differ from our current tripartite clinical categorization. More important, these biological stages might eventually be associated with differential responses to current or future medication regimens. These issues open an entire field of new research questions, but first, the cross-sectional and longitudinal studies in AD must be carried out to establish the "norms" for these biomarkers over the course of the illness. Paradoxically, the fact that our current clinical medications are relatively ineffective in slowing the course of AD may allow for these biomarkers to be better studied over the next few years in anticipation of future medications that are more pathophysiologically relevant and effective. This research would lay the groundwork for a more distinct and biologically relevant clinical staging of AD once the diagnosis was established and intervention strategies are planned.

Biomarkers as a Prognostic Measure of Alzheimer's Disease Risk

Generally, clinicians focus on the confirmation of the AD diagnosis only when individuals have already manifested specific cognitive complaints. Most of our prior discussion has followed that line of thinking, especially because the diagnosis of AD is currently defined as a cognitive disorder. In fact, all of our existing nomenclature requires evidence of cognitive impairment before the diagnosis can be entertained (Table 7–1). Even mild cognitive impairment (MCI), considered by many to be an early or transitional presentation of AD with its own distinct clinical characteristics (see Chapter 4 by Dr. Petersen and O'Brien in this volume), is defined by cognitive manifestations. But AD is a neuropsychiatric disorder with known neuropathological characteristics.[38] Assuming that biomarkers are eventually established as a routine part of the clinical diagnosis of AD, it is not difficult to imagine how they will soon be applied to normal control participants as potential prognostic measures of AD.[39–42] Not surprisingly, there is already a growing literature on biomarkers associated with the transition of MCI to AD (Table 7–3).

Whereas the clinical correlates for biomarkers in MCI and AD are obvious (i.e., cognitive testing), there are no such clinical correlates in asymptomatic individuals who may be "at risk" for eventually developing dementia. Therefore, the study of biomarkers as prognostic risk factors for AD becomes, by definition, a longitudinal process. Even if AD-like patterns of biomarkers are discovered in any such population, proven conversion of these potential endophenotypes to more classic phenotypes of MCI or AD with cognitive manifestations is most likely required before scientists and clinicians will be convinced of the prognostic value of these patterns. These studies are expensive, time-consuming, and high risk scientifically, but the potential benefit is enormous if a biological precursor to AD can be illuminated and chronicled longitudinally. Currently, a small number of such studies are going on internationally,[22,39,43–45] but this area of research is still in development.

TABLE 7–3.   Measures suggested as predictors of conversion from mild cognitive impairment to Alzheimer's disease

Category	Selected markers	References
Cognitive tests	Word recall, associate learning, category fluency, and mental speed	67–71
Brain imaging	EEG, CT, MRI, atrophy rates, diffusion-weighted MRI, SPECT, PET, fMRI, and combination of MRI and SPECT	67, 72–78
Cerebrospinal fluid	β-amyloid$_{1-42}$, β-amyloid$_{1-40}$, total tau, p-tau, other β-amyloid peptides, and combinations of CSF peptides	22, 32, 40, 41, 79–82
Combination approaches	Neuropsychological tests and *APOE* ϵ4, memory testing and brain atrophy, memory testing and CSF peptides, CSF peptides and brain imaging	42, 73, 83–85

Note.   *APOE* = apolipoprotein E gene; CSF = cerebrospinal fluid; CT = computed tomography; EEG = electroencephalography; fMRI = functional MRI; MRI = magnetic resonance imaging; PET = positron emission tomography; SPECT = single photon emission computed tomography.

Conclusion

The effort to develop diagnostic and prognostic measures has enormous implications for our nomenclature and future clinical practices. If and when a recognizable and reproducible pattern of biological changes emerges as characteristic of AD, MCI, or pre-MCI, then we have to question our current reliance on clinical manifestations as the main diagnostic anchors for the illness. Always keeping in mind the profound importance of the available therapeutic options that will (or will not) drive the clinical interest in this phenomenon, we may theoretically soon face the situation where we can diagnose an AD-like condition in seemingly normal-functioning individuals long before there is any clinical (i.e., cognitive) manifestation of the illness. How will this happen? It is unlikely that the diagnostic specificity and sensitivity data in prognostic studies will approach the 85%–90% levels seen

TABLE 7–4. Suggested future directions in biomarker diagnostic research

Development of longitudinal CSF biomarker specimen bank

Acquisition of CSF specimens for all stages of AD cross-sectionally

Comparison of CSF biomarkers with concurrent brain biopsy specimens

Comparison of CSF biomarkers with simultaneous brain imaging

Development of consistent, reliable tests for individual biomarkers

Correlation of biomarkers with clinical parameters longitudinally

Drug studies in AD patients using biomarkers as dependent variables

Conversion studies using biomarkers as predictors of control to MCI to AD

Note. AD=Alzheimer's disease; CSF=cerebrospinal fluid; MCI=mild cognitive impairment.

currently with these biomarkers in comparisons of well-characterized AD patients versus control populations. Nonetheless, lower levels of specificity and sensitivity may be sufficient to establish prognostic likelihoods or risk estimates, especially when combined with genetic profiles or other risk factors, and some suggested future directions are summarized in Table 7–4. As was the case in general medicine with certain types of hepatitis or HIV infection before the advent of antiretroviral medications, neuropsychiatry may soon be faced with the difficult reality of vastly improved diagnostic certainty or predictability of AD long before there are acceptable therapeutic options. In the meantime, multiple legal, ethical, and counseling issues could be addressed in these situations that would be of immense clinical value, even in the absence of proven therapeutic options.

When the National Institute on Aging consensus conference met in 1998 to define the ideal characteristics of a diagnostic marker, the participants cited ease of use, simplicity, and low cost as three practical characteristics.[27] Although each of these is an important target goal, none is essential if the diagnostic data are compelling. Although brain biopsy is not likely ever to be considered noninvasive, simple to perform, or inexpensive, it could theoretically become a routine procedure if it met all the other criteria listed (related, valid, specific, and reliable), it was the only such procedure available, and the certain diagnosis of AD or pre-AD was associated with a significant therapeutic advantage. For instance, if it were proven that a certain level of β-amyloid deposition in the temporal cortex of a normal patient on biopsy was highly associated with AD in 2–3 years and that early intervention with a (yet-to-be-determined) β-amyloid prevention agent would significantly delay or prevent AD, then the biopsy procedure would take on a new light. The morbidity associated with the biopsy would have to be considered alongside the potential advantage of the clinical intervention proposed. As a result, this intervention eventually might be considered equivalent to the exploratory colonoscopy now commonly recommended for people over 50 years of age to diagnose and prevent the spread of in situ colon cancer.[46] Less invasive measures of β-amyloid buildup quantification such as brain positron emission tomography scan quantification of PIB would be another possible clinical advance, but, like virtual colonoscopy imaging,[47] PIB PET or some imaging equivalent would eventually have to be proven of similar value in the diagnostic process by comparison with biopsy or autopsy data. Thus, the science of biomarkers still has room to grow before it significantly alters the diagnostic nomenclature for dementia, but that time is rapidly approaching and may already be here for some of the CSF measures of β-amyloid and tau.

References

1. Maltoni M, Caraceni A, Brunelli C, et al: Prognostic factors in advanced cancer patients: evidence-based clinical recommendations—a study by the Steering Committee of the European Association for Palliative Care. J Clin Oncol 23:6240–6248, 2005.
2. Miller PD: Bone density and markers of bone turnover in predicting fracture risk and how changes in these measures predict fracture risk reduction. Curr Osteoporos Rep 3:103–110, 2005.
3. Sunderland T, Gur RE, Arnold SE: The use of biomarkers in the elderly: current and future challenges. Biol Psychiatry 58:272–276, 2005.
4. Mirra SS, Heyman A, McKeel D, et al: The Consortium to Establish a Registry for Alzheimer's Disease (CERAD), Part II: standardization of the neuropathologic assessment of Alzheimer's disease. Neurology 41:479–486, 1991.
5. Mendez MF, Mastri AR, Sung JH, et al: Clinically diagnosed Alzheimer disease: neuropathologic findings in 650 cases. Alzheimer Dis Assoc Disord 6:35–43, 1992.
6. McKhann G, Drachman D, Folstein M, et al: Clinical diagnosis of Alzheimer's disease: report of the NINCDS-ADRDA Work Group under the auspices of Department of Health and Human Services Task Force on Alzheimer's Disease. Neurology 34:939–944, 1984.
7. World Health Organization: The ICD-10 Classification of Mental and Behavioural Disorders: Clinical Descriptions and Diagnostic Guidelines. Geneva, World Health Organization, 1992.
8. American Psychiatric Association: Diagnostic and Statistical Manual of Mental Disorders, 4th Edition, Text Revision. Washington, DC, American Psychiatric Association, 2000.
9. Lim A, Tsuang D, Kukull W, et al: Clinico-neuropathological correlation of Alzheimer's disease in a community-based case series. J Am Geriatr Soc 47:564–569, 1999.
10. Newell KL, Hyman BT, Growdon JH, et al: Application of the National Institute on Aging (NIA)–Reagan Institute criteria for the neuropathologic diagnosis of Alzheimer disease. J Neuropathol Exp Neurol 58:1147–1155, 1999.
11. Plassman BL, Khachaturian AS, Townsend JJ, et al: Comparison of clinical and neuropathologic diagnoses of Alzheimer's disease in three epidemiologic samples. Alzheimer's & Dementia 2:2–11, 2006.
12. Lopez OL, Becker JT, Kaufer DI, et al: Research evaluation and prospective diagnosis of dementia with Lewy bodies. Arch Neurol 59:43–46, 2002.
13. Scinto LF, Daffner KR, Dressler D, et al: A potential noninvasive neurobiological test for Alzheimer's disease. Science 266:1051–1054, 1994.

14. Arai H, Terajima M, Miura M, et al: Tau in cerebrospinal fluid: a potential diagnostic marker in Alzheimer's disease. Ann Neurol 38:649–652, 1995.
15. Small GW, Komo S, La Rue A, et al: Early detection of Alzheimer's disease by combining apolipoprotein E and neuroimaging. Ann N Y Acad Sci 802:70–78, 1996.
16. Jack CR Jr, Petersen RC, Xu YC, et al: Medial temporal atrophy on MRI in normal aging and very mild Alzheimer's disease. Neurology 49:786–794, 1997.
17. Andreasen N, Minthon L, Clarberg A, et al: Sensitivity, specificity, and stability of CSF-tau in AD in a community-based patient sample. Neurology 53:1488–1494, 1999.
18. Blennow K, Vanmechelen E, Hampel H: CSF total tau, Abeta42 and phosphorylated tau protein as biomarkers for Alzheimer's disease. Mol Neurobiol 24:87–97, 2001.
19. Seshadri S, Beiser A, Selhub J, et al: Plasma homocysteine as a risk factor for dementia and Alzheimer's disease. N Engl J Med 346:476–483, 2002.
20. Munzar M, Levy S, Rush R, et al: Clinical study of a urinary competitive ELISA for neural thread protein in Alzheimer disease. Neurol Clin Neurophysiol 2002(1):2–8, 2002.
21. Sunderland T, Linker G, Mirza N, et al: Decreased beta-amyloid$_{1-42}$ and increased tau levels in cerebrospinal fluid of patients with Alzheimer disease. JAMA 289:2094–2103, 2003.
22. Hampel H, Teipel SJ, Fuchsberger T, et al: Value of CSF beta-amyloid$_{1-42}$ and tau as predictors of Alzheimer's disease in patients with mild cognitive impairment. Mol Psychiatry 9:705–710, 2004.
23. Francis PT, Palmer AM, Sims NR, et al: Neurochemical studies of early-onset Alzheimer's disease. Possible influence on treatment. N Engl J Med 313:7–11, 1985.
24. Mayeux R, Tang MX, Jacobs DM, et al: Plasma amyloid beta-peptide$_{1-42}$ and incipient Alzheimer's disease. Ann Neurol 46:412–416, 1999.
25. Mehta PD, Pirttila T, Patrick BA, et al: Amyloid beta protein 1–40 and 1–42 levels in matched cerebrospinal fluid and plasma from patients with Alzheimer disease. Neurosci Lett 304:102–106, 2001.
26. Galasko D, Chang L, Motter R, et al: High cerebrospinal fluid tau and low amyloid beta42 levels in the clinical diagnosis of Alzheimer disease and relation to apolipoprotein E genotype. Arch Neurol 55:937–945, 1998.
27. Consensus report of the Working Group on: "Molecular and Biochemical Markers of Alzheimer's Disease." The Ronald and Nancy Reagan Research Institute of the Alzheimer's Association and the National Institute on Aging Working Group. Neurobiol Aging 19:109–116, 1998.
28. Galasko D: CSF tau and Abeta42: logical biomarkers for Alzheimer's disease? Neurobiol Aging 19:117–119, 1998.
29. Blennow K, Hampel H: CSF markers for incipient Alzheimer's disease. Lancet Neurol 2:605–613, 2003.
30. Wiltfang J, Lewczuk P, Riederer P, et al: Consensus paper of the WFSBP Task Force on Biological Markers of Dementia: the role of CSF and blood analysis in the early and differential diagnosis of dementia. World J Biol Psychiatry 6:69–84, 2005.
31. Mitchell A, Brindle N: CSF phosphorylated tau—does it constitute an accurate biological test for Alzheimer's disease? Int J Geriatr Psychiatry 18:407–411, 2003.

32. Buerger K, Zinkowski R, Teipel SJ, et al: Differential diagnosis of Alzheimer disease with cerebrospinal fluid levels of tau protein phosphorylated at threonine 231. Arch Neurol 59:1267–1272, 2002.

33. Hampel H, Buerger K, Zinkowski R, et al: Measurement of phosphorylated tau epitopes in the differential diagnosis of Alzheimer disease: a comparative cerebrospinal fluid study. Arch Gen Psychiatry 61:95–102, 2004.

34. Klunk WE, Engler H, Nordberg A, et al: Imaging brain amyloid in Alzheimer's disease with Pittsburgh Compound-B. Ann Neurol 55:306–319, 2004.

35. Linker G, Mirza N, Manetti G, et al: Fine-needle, negative-pressure lumbar puncture: a safe technique for collecting CSF. Neurology 59:2008–2009, 2002.

36. Peskind ER, Riekse R, Quinn JF, et al: Safety and acceptability of the research lumbar puncture. Alzheimer Dis Assoc Disord 19:220–225, 2005.

37. Hughes CP, Berg L, Danziger WL, et al: A new clinical scale for the staging of dementia. Br J Psychiatry 140:566–572, 1982.

38. Petersen RC, Smith GE, Waring SC, et al: Mild cognitive impairment: clinical characterization and outcome. Arch Neurol 56:303–308, 1999.

39. Sunderland T, Mirza N, Putnam KT, et al: Cerebrospinal fluid beta-amyloid1-42 and tau in control subjects at risk for Alzheimer's disease: the effect of APOE epsilon4 allele. Biol Psychiatry 56:670–676, 2004.

40. Herukka SK, Helisalmi S, Hallikainen M, et al: CSF Abeta42, Tau and phosphorylated Tau, APOE varepsilon4 allele and MCI type in progressive MCI. Neurobiol Aging March 17, 2006 [epub ahead of print].

41. Hansson O, Zetterberg H, Buchhave P, et al: Association between CSF biomarkers and incipient Alzheimer's disease in patients with mild cognitive impairment: a follow-up study. Lancet Neurol 5:228–234, 2006.

42. de Leon MJ, DeSanti S, Zinkowski R, et al: Longitudinal CSF and MRI biomarkers improve the diagnosis of mild cognitive impairment. Neurobiol Aging 27:394–401, 2006.

43. Andreasen N, Vanmechelen E, Vanderstichele H, et al: Cerebrospinal fluid levels of total-tau, phospho-tau and Abeta 42 predicts development of Alzheimer's disease in patients with mild cognitive impairment. Acta Neurol Scand Suppl 179:47–51, 2003.

44. Mueller SG, Weiner MW, Thal LJ, et al: The Alzheimer's Disease Neuroimaging Initiative. Neuroimaging Clin N Am 15:869–877, xi–xii, 2005.

45. Sager MA, Hermann B, La Rue A: Middle-aged children of persons with Alzheimer's disease: APOE genotypes and cognitive function in the Wisconsin Registry for Alzheimer's Prevention. J Geriatr Psychiatry Neurol 18:245–249, 2005.

46. Hilsden RJ, McGregor E, Murray A, et al: Colorectal cancer screening: practices and attitudes of gastroenterologists, internists and surgeons. Can J Surg 48:434–440, 2005.

47. O'Hare A, Fenlon H: Virtual colonoscopy in the detection of colonic polyps and neoplasms. Best Pract Res Clin Gastroenterol 20:79–92, 2006.

48. Smyth MD, Cribbs DH, Tenner AJ, et al: Decreased levels of C1q in cerebrospinal fluid of living Alzheimer patients correlate with disease state. Neurobiol Aging 15:609–614, 1994.

49. Papassotiropoulos A, Lutjohann D, Bagli M, et al: 24S-Hydroxycholesterol in cerebrospinal fluid is elevated in early stages of dementia. J Psychiatr Res 36:27–32, 2002.

50. Bretillon L, Siden A,Wahlund LO, et al: Plasma levels of 24S-hydroxycholesterol in patients with neurological diseases. Neurosci Lett 293:87–90, 2000.

51. Morris MS, Jacques PF, Rosenberg IH, et al: Hyperhomocysteinemia associated with poor recall in the third National Health and Nutrition Examination Survey. Am J Clin Nutr 73:927–933, 2001.

52. Pratico D, Clark CM, Lee VM, et al: Increased 8,12-iso-iPF2alpha-VI in Alzheimer's disease: correlation of a noninvasive index of lipid peroxidation with disease severity. Ann Neurol 48:809–812, 2000.

53. Grossman M, Farmer J, Leight S, et al: Cerebrospinal fluid profile in frontotemporal dementia and Alzheimer's disease. Ann Neurol 57:721–729, 2005.

54. Licastro F, Pedrini S, Caputo L, et al: Increased plasma levels of interleukin-1, interleukin-6 and alpha-1-antichymotrypsin in patients with Alzheimer's disease: peripheral inflammation or signals from the brain? J Neuroimmunol 103:97–102, 2000.

55. Jobst KA, Barnetson LP, Shepstone BJ: Accurate prediction of histologically confirmed Alzheimer's disease and the differential diagnosis of dementia: the use of NINCDS-ADRDA and DSM-III-R criteria, SPECT, X-ray CT, and Apo E4 in medial temporal lobe dementias. Oxford Project to Investigate Memory and Aging. Int Psychogeriatr 10:271–302, 1998.

56. Nagy Z, Hindley NJ, Braak H, et al: Relationship between clinical and radiological diagnostic criteria for Alzheimer's disease and the extent of neuropathology as reflected by "stages": a prospective study. Dement Geriatr Cogn Disord 10:109–114, 1999.

57. Fox NC, Schott JM: Imaging cerebral atrophy: normal ageing to Alzheimer's disease. Lancet 363:392–394, 2004.

58. Jack CR Jr, Dickson DW, Parisi JE, et al: Antemortem MRI findings correlate with hippocampal neuropathology in typical aging and dementia. Neurology 58:750–757, 2002.

59. Verhoeff NP, Wilson AA, Takeshita S, et al: In-vivo imaging of Alzheimer disease beta-amyloid with [11C]SB-13 PET. Am J Geriatr Psychiatry 12:584–595, 2004.

60. Bokde AL, Lopez-Bayo P, Meindl T, et al: Functional connectivity of the fusiform gyrus during a face-matching task in subjects with mild cognitive impairment. Brain 129:1113–1124, 2006.

61. Sunderland T, Wolozin B, Galasko D, et al: Longitudinal stability of CSF tau levels in Alzheimer patients. Biol Psychiatry 46:750–755, 1999.

62. Sjogren M, Vanderstichele H, Agren H, et al: Tau and Abeta42 in cerebrospinal fluid from healthy adults 21–93 years of age: establishment of reference values. Clin Chem 47:1776–1781, 2001.

63. Hampel H, Teipel SJ, Fuchsberger T, et al: Value of CSF beta-amyloid$_{1-42}$ and tau as predictors of Alzheimer's disease in patients with mild cognitive impairment. Mol Psychiatry 9:705–710, 2004.

64. Motter R, Vigo-Pelfrey C, Kholodenko D, et al: Reduction of beta-amyloid peptide42 in the cerebrospinal fluid of patients with Alzheimer's disease. Ann Neurol 38:643–648, 1995.

65. Arai H: Biological markers for the clinical diagnosis of Alzheimer's disease. Tohoku J Exp Med 179:65–79, 1996.

66. Buerger K, Teipel SJ, Zinkowski R, et al: CSF tau protein phosphorylated at threonine 231 correlates with cognitive decline in MCI subjects. Neurology 59:627–629, 2002.

67. De Jager CA, Hogervorst E, Combrinck M, et al: Sensitivity and specificity of neuro-psychological tests for mild cognitive impairment, vascular cognitive impairment and Alzheimer's disease. Psychol Med 33:1039–1050, 2003.

68. Nestor PJ, Scheltens P, Hodges JR: Advances in the early detection of Alzheimer's disease. Nat Med 10(suppl):S34–S41, 2004.

69. DeCarli C, Mungas D, Harvey D, et al: Memory impairment, but not cerebrovascular disease, predicts progression of MCI to dementia. Neurology 63:220–227, 2004.

70. Amieva H, Letenneur L, Dartigues JF, et al: Annual rate and predictors of conversion to dementia in subjects presenting mild cognitive impairment criteria defined according to a population-based study. Dement Geriatr Cogn Disord 18:87–93, 2004.

71. Greenwood PM, Lambert C, Sunderland T, et al: Effects of apolipoprotein E genotype on spatial attention, working memory, and their interaction in healthy, middle-aged adults: results from the National Institute of Mental Health's BIOCARD study. Neuropsychology 19:199–211, 2005.

72. Jelic V, Johansson SE, Almkvist O, et al: Quantitative electroencephalography in mild cognitive impairment: longitudinal changes and possible prediction of Alzheimer's disease. Neurobiol Aging 21:533–540, 2000.

73. Arnaiz E, Jelic V, Almkvist O, et al: Impaired cerebral glucose metabolism and cognitive functioning predict deterioration in mild cognitive impairment. Neuroreport 12:851–855, 2001.

74. Visser PJ, Verhey FR, Hofman PA, et al: Medial temporal lobe atrophy predicts Alzheimer's disease in patients with minor cognitive impairment. J Neurol Neurosurg Psychiatry 72:491–497, 2002.

75. Chetelat G, Desgranges B, de la Sayette V, et al: Mild cognitive impairment: can FDG-PET predict who is to rapidly convert to Alzheimer's disease? Neurology 60:1374–1377, 2003.

76. deToledo-Morrell L, Stoub TR, Bulgakova M, et al: MRI-derived entorhinal volume is a good predictor of conversion from MCI to AD. Neurobiol Aging 25:1197–1203, 2004.

77. Korf ES, Wahlund LO, Visser PJ, et al: Medial temporal lobe atrophy on MRI predicts dementia in patients with mild cognitive impairment. Neurology 63:94–100, 2004.

78. Jack CR Jr, Shiung MM, Weigand SD, et al: Brain atrophy rates predict subsequent clinical conversion in normal elderly and amnestic MCI. Neurology 65:1227–1231, 2005.

79. Arai H, Terajima M, Miura M, et al: Effect of genetic risk factors and disease progression on the cerebrospinal fluid tau levels in Alzheimer's disease. J Am Geriatr Soc 45:1228–1231, 1997.

80. Arai H, Ishiguro K, Ohno H, et al: CSF phosphorylated tau protein and mild cognitive impairment: a prospective study. Exp Neurol 166:201–203, 2000.

81. Riemenschneider M, Lautenschlager N, Wagenpfeil S, et al: Cerebrospinal fluid tau and beta-amyloid 42 proteins identify Alzheimer disease in subjects with mild cognitive impairment. Arch Neurol 59:1729–1734, 2002.

82. Vanderstichele H, De Meyer G, Andreasen N, et al: Amino-truncated beta-amyloid$_{42}$ peptides in cerebrospinal fluid and prediction of progression of mild cognitive impairment. Clin Chem 51:1650–1660, 2005.

83. Okamura N, Arai H, Maruyama M, et al: Combined analysis of CSF tau levels and [(123)I]iodoamphetamine SPECT in mild cognitive impairment: implications for a novel predictor of Alzheimer's disease. Am J Psychiatry 159:474–476, 2002.

84. El Fakhri G, Kijewski MF, Johnson KA, et al: MRI-guided SPECT perfusion measures and volumetric MRI in prodromal Alzheimer disease. Arch Neurol 60:1066–1072, 2003.
85. Dickerson BC, Salat DH, Bates JF, et al: Medial temporal lobe function and structure in mild cognitive impairment. Ann Neurol 56:27–35, 2004.

8

NEUROIMAGING AS A SURROGATE MARKER OF DISEASE

Gary W. Small, M.D.

The risk for cognitive decline increases with age. When such decline interferes with daily functioning, a diagnosis of dementia is generally present. Alzheimer's disease (AD), the most common cause of dementia, afflicts 10% or more of people age 65 years and older and accounts for the most striking increase in dementia incidence in the very old.[1,2] Characterized by deterioration in memory, language, behavior, and ability to function, AD is a chronic disorder that eventually necessitates total care.

The neuropathological hallmarks of AD, amyloid neuritic plaques (NPs) and neurofibrillary tangles (NFTs), have been found in older people with memory impairment too mild to justify a diagnosis of dementia, such as mild cognitive impairment (MCI).[3] Amnestic MCI is characterized by memory loss that is not associated with functional decline. Approximately 10% of people 65 years of age or older suffer from MCI, and an estimated 15% of those with amnestic MCI will develop AD each year.[4,5]

Loss of caregiver productivity, increased medical expenses, and long-term as well as short-term care lead to annual estimated costs of AD approaching $100 bil-

This chapter is reprinted from Small GW: "Diagnostic Issues in Dementia: Neuroimaging as a Surrogate Marker of Disease." *Journal of Geriatric Psychiatry and Neurology* 19:180–185, 2006. Used with permission.

lion in the United States alone.[6,7] The total cost, both financial and emotional, of diagnosing and managing patients with dementia and other age-related cognitive deficits presents a major challenge to the medical community as well as to society.

Diagnosis of Dementia

The clinical presentation of gradually progressive cognitive decline presents a clinical challenge because it can be difficult to differentiate from normal aging. Differential diagnosis among the various dementias, including dementia with Lewy bodies, frontotemporal dementia (FTD), vascular dementia, and dementia syndrome of depression, is an additional challenge. Differentiating FTD from AD is important because FTD patients appear to respond poorly to currently available drugs for AD. In milder dementia states, this diagnostic challenge is further complicated in attempts to differentiate MCI from AD and other forms of dementia. Although these conditions can be differentiated in research settings,[8] in clinical practice the diagnosis is often missed. Physicians often fail to correctly apply a diagnosis of dementia, making a positive diagnosis when the disease is not present or failing to recognize it when it is present.[9,10] Because treatment benefit is likely in the early stages of disease, investigators have focused on developing tools for earlier detection to identify treatment candidates in the milder phases of age-related cognitive decline.

Genetic testing is not routinely used in the assessment of dementia, but it can be helpful for rare familial cases and in research of individuals at risk for dementia. Mutations on chromosomes 1, 14, and 21 are associated with early onset of the extremely rare, familial form of AD.[2] The *APOE* ε4 allele on chromosome 19 is associated with a dose-related risk increase for typical AD, which begins after the age of 60 years.[11,12] The isoforms of *APOE* include *APOE* ε2, *APOE* ε3, and *APOE* ε4. Forty percent of sporadic, late-onset AD patients have the *APOE* ε4 allele, whereas *APOE* ε3 is the most common allele in the general population. The risk of developing AD increases eight times if two copies of *APOE* ε4 are inherited compared with two copies of *APOE* ε3. Use of the *APOE* ε4 allele to assist in the prediction of cognitive decline is not recommended, because the allele is found in elderly persons without AD, and many patients with the disease do not have the allele.[13,14] However, combining *APOE* genetic data with other relevant biological information from neuroimaging studies has proved to be a useful strategy for early detection of subtle brain abnormalities.

Structural Imaging

The most recent practice parameter guidelines from the American Academy of Neurology recommended the routine use of structural neuroimaging studies (either computed tomography or magnetic resonance imaging [MRI]) to assist with the diagnosis of dementia. In clinical settings, such structural studies can identify evidence of stroke or a space-occupying lesion, but findings of general atrophy and white matter changes are nonspecific and do not assist in the differential diagnosis.[15] Early neuropathological changes in AD include the formation of NFTs first in the entorhinal cortex and then the hippocampus,[16] and structural imaging studies in research centers have noted atrophy in such medial temporal regions in patients with AD.[17] In older MCI patients, hippocampal atrophy may predict subsequent conversion to AD.[18] Structural MRI in older patients without cognitive deficits may show medial temporal atrophy, suggesting the possibility of future cognitive decline; however, a significant portion of neural cell death is necessary before cerebral atrophy is visualized, which may limit structural imaging as the optimal means for early diagnosis.

Functional Imaging

Although single photon emission computed tomography has been a widely available method of functional brain imaging, its spatial resolution is lower than that of positron emission tomography (PET). In 2004, the Centers for Medicare and Medicaid Services made PET using ^{18}F-fluorodeoxyglucose (FDG) available to Medicare recipients to assist with the diagnosis of dementia when both AD and FTD are being considered. Studies of regional glucose metabolic rates using FDG-PET imaging show that in AD, metabolic deficits are present in the neocortical association areas, with sparing of the basal ganglia, thalamus, cerebellum, and the primary sensory and motor cortex.[19] Decreased metabolic rates are typically observed in the temporal and parietal regions in AD, and the extent of the hypometabolism has correlated with the severity of cognitive impairment.[20]

Typical PET metabolic patterns are observed for dementia with Lewy bodies (temporal, parietal, occipital, and cerebellar deficits),[21,22] FTD (frontal deficits),[23] Huntington's dementia (caudate deficits),[24] and Parkinson's dementia (parietal, frontal, lateral temporal, and visual cortical deficits).[25]

Studies indicate that PET provides greater diagnostic accuracy when compared with clinical assessments without functional imaging. Our group[26] studied FDG-PET scans in 146 patients undergoing evaluation for dementia with at least 2 years of follow-up and 138 patients with histopathological diagnoses an average of 2.9 years later. Among patients with neuropathologically based diagnoses, PET identified patients with AD and patients with any neurodegenerative disease with a sensitivity of 94% and specificities of 73% and 78%, respectively. The initial pattern of cerebral metabolism was significantly associated with the subsequent course of progression overall ($P < .001$). In patients presenting with cognitive symptoms of dementia, regional brain metabolism was a sensitive indicator of AD and of neurodegenerative disease in general. A negative PET scan indicated that pathological progression of cognitive impairment during the mean 3-year follow-up was unlikely to occur.

Standardized metabolic reductions using three-dimensional stereotactic surface projections from FDG-PET scans of AD patients compared with controls also provide a high degree of accuracy, yielding a sensitivity as high as 97% when specificity is set at 100%.[27] A study comparing FDG-PET patterns of 10 MCI patients who converted to dementia within 18 months with 7 nonconverters found that all converters demonstrated lower FDG uptake in temporal parietal cortex.[28]

Studies of asymptomatic members of families that have a history of AD also show significant temporal and parietal hypometabolism relative to normal control participants.[29] Furthermore, middle-aged participants who do not have dementia but who have a genetic risk for AD because of the presence of the *APOE* ε4 allele have significantly lower temporal, parietal, and posterior cingulate metabolism than those without the allele.[20,30]

To determine cognitive and metabolic decline patterns according to genetic risk, our group[31] investigated cerebral metabolic rates using PET in middle-aged and older nondemented persons with normal memory performance. A single copy of the APOE ε4 allele was associated with lowered inferior parietal, lateral temporal, and posterior cingulate metabolism, which predicted cognitive decline after 2 years of longitudinal follow-up. For the 20 nondemented participants followed longitudinally, memory performance scores did not decline significantly but cortical metabolic rates did. In APOE ε4 carriers, a 4% left posterior cingulate metabolic decline was observed, and inferior parietal and lateral temporal regions demonstrated the greatest magnitude (5%) of metabolic decline after 2 years. Reiman and associates[32] confirmed these findings in independent samples.

These results have practical implications for clinical trials of dementia prevention treatments. For example, the right lateral temporal metabolism for APOE ε4 carriers at baseline and 2-year follow-up yielded an estimated power under the most conservative scenario (i.e., assuming that the points are connected exactly in reverse order) of .9 to detect a one-unit decline from baseline to follow-up using a one-tailed test.[31] A sample size of only 20 participants, therefore, would be needed in each treatment arm (i.e., active drug or placebo) to detect a drug-effect size of .8 (α=.05, power=.8). Thus, a clinical trial of a novel intervention to prevent cerebral metabolic decline would require only 40 participants over a 2-year treatment period. Such findings suggest that combining PET and AD genetic risk measures would allow investigators to use relatively small sample sizes when testing treatments for preventing cognitive decline in participants with mild age-related memory complaints. These results indicate that the combination of cerebral metabolic rates and genetic risk factors provides a means for presymptomatic AD detection that will assist in response monitoring during experimental treatments.

Acetylcholine, a neurotransmitter important to memory and attention, has reduced concentrations in AD cerebral cortex. Cholinesterase inhibitors were developed to increase brain acetylcholine levels and thus improve cognitive performance. These drugs work by inhibiting acetylcholinesterase or butyrylcholinesterase or both, enzymes that hydrolyze acetylcholine. Double-blind placebo-controlled trials of these drugs have shown that they improve cognition and function compared with placebo.[2] When investigators use FDG-PET as a surrogate marker during such treatment trials, they find that cholinesterase inhibition stabilizes metabolism in parietal and frontal regions.[33]

Including a task during functional imaging can provide additional information. For example, Bookheimer and colleagues[34] studied 30 cognitively intact older adults for patterns in brain activation in response to a memory task. Scan results were analyzed according to genetic risk so that *APOE* ε4 carriers were compared with noncarriers. The left hippocampal, parietal, and prefrontal regions, areas typically affected by AD, exhibited greater magnitude and extent of activation during word recall in *APOE* ε4 carriers compared with noncarriers. Participants with the *APOE* ε4 genetic risk also had a greater average increase in signal intensity in the hippocampus and a greater number of activated regions than did noncarriers during periods of recall.

Memory performance scores obtained 2 years after the baseline scans indicated that the degree of baseline brain activation correlated with the degree of memory decline. These results suggest that increased brain activity among *APOE* ε4 carriers reflects a compensatory cognitive response to subtle brain deficits attributable to genetic risk. The presence of adequate amounts of healthy neural tissue is necessary for signal intensity to increase in association with compensatory processing. Therefore, neuronal loss as is found in AD would be associated with attenuated brain activity.

In Vivo Neuroimaging of Amyloid Neuritic Plaques and Neurofibrillary Tangles

The evidence for NP and NFT accumulation years before clinical AD diagnosis suggests that in vivo methods that directly image these pathognomonic lesions would be useful presymptomatic detection technologies. Most current methods for measuring brain amyloid, such as histochemical stains, require tissue fixation on postmortem or biopsy material. Most available in vivo methods for measuring NPs or NFTs are indirect (e.g., cerebrospinal fluid measures). Studies that may lead to direct in vivo human Aβ imaging include various radiolabeled probes using small organic and organometallic molecules capable of detecting differences in amyloid fibril structure or amyloid protein sequences.[35] Investigators also have used chrysamine-G, a carboxylic acid analogue of Congo red; an amyloid-staining histologic dye[36];

serum amyloid P component, a normal plasma glycoprotein that binds to amyloid deposit fibrils[37]; or monoclonal antibodies.[38] Methodological difficulties that hinder progress with these techniques include poor blood–brain barrier crossing and limited specificity and sensitivity. In addition, most approaches do not measure both NPs and NFTs.

Only recently have scientists been able to provide measures of NPs and NFTs in the living patient. Our group has developed a small molecule, 2-(1-{6-[(2-[F-18]-fluoroethyl)(methyl)amino]-2-naphthyl}ethylidene)malononitrile (FDDNP), for use as an in vivo chemical marker of these abnormal brain protein aggregates. After intravenous FDDNP injection, PET scans show significantly higher FDDNP binding in temporal, parietal, and frontal brain regions in AD patients compared with older, cognitively intact controls.[39] Both FDDNP and its parent molecule, DDNP, are fluorescent and provide clear in vitro visualizations of plaques and tangles in Alzheimer's brain specimens examined under a confocal fluorescence microscope.[40]

Previous PET studies have found differences in cerebral amyloid measures, using FDDNP or other amyloid imaging tracers such as Pittsburgh Compound B, when small groups of dementia patients and controls are compared.[39,41,42] Our group[43] recently reported that FDDNP-PET may differentiate normal cognitively intact older adults from patients with MCI or AD. We performed PET scans on subjects after intravenous injections of FDDNP, and scans were repeated for nine participants (five controls, four MCI participants) after approximately 2 years. Autopsy follow-up was available on one patient with AD. Global FDDNP-PET binding (temporal, parietal, posterior cingulate, and frontal average) was lower for the control group compared with the MCI group, which showed lower binding compared with the AD group. At follow-up, participants who converted from normal cognitive status to MCI or from MCI to AD showed regional FDDNP binding increases, and autopsy follow-up demonstrated high concentrations of plaques and tangles in brain regions with high FDDNP binding.

Several potential therapeutic strategies for preventing or diminishing insoluble amyloid accumulation—such as secretase inhibitors or modulators, active or passive vaccines, anti-inflammatory drugs, and the yellow curry pigment, curcumin—are being explored as interventions for delaying onset or slowing progression of AD. Our initial results suggest that FDDNP-PET may serve as a useful surrogate marker of the efficacy of such treatments designed to lower the concentration of plaques. Investigators could focus on tangle-sparse and amyloid-rich brain regions when testing antiplaque treatments. As additional treatments targeting cerebral tauopathies emerge, FDDNP-PET may also provide a surrogate measure of antitangle treatments in tangle-rich, medial temporal brain regions. Our group has found that microPET studies demonstrate high FDDNP binding in hippocampus and frontal cortex in transgenic amyloid rat models of AD.[44] These same transgenic animals show minimal FDDNP binding after 2 days of treatment with the nonsteroidal anti-inflammatory drug naproxen, a competitive inhibitor of FDDNP binding,[45] thus demonstrating high in vivo specificity of FDDNP binding. These experiments provide a proof of concept for an antiplaque/antitangle drug discovery strategy: initial testing of compounds in animal models followed by small animal studies using FDDNP-microPET as the surrogate marker, to guide investigators on further testing in humans, using FDDNP-PET as the surrogate marker.

Need for Revised Diagnostic Considerations

The current version of the *Diagnostic and Statistical Manual of Mental Disorders*[46] mentions imaging in the associated laboratory findings section of the dementia chapter. This section needs to be updated and expanded to include some of the aforementioned points regarding the use of imaging in diagnosis and differential diagnosis, as well as its emerging use as a surrogate marker of disease and treatment response. For example, FDG-PET has become increasingly available since policy makers approved it for Medicare funding to assist in the diagnosis of dementia. In addition to expanding some of this information in the appropriate paragraph, some mention of imaging as a diagnostic tool would be appropriate for the diagnostic criteria section (e.g., "The diagnosis of AD is supported by the presence of parietal–temporal hypometabolism on FDG-PET scans" and "The diagnosis of FTD is supported by the presence of frontal-temporal hypometabolism on FDG-PET scans"). For the section on MCI, imaging information is appropriate as well. As noted, recent studies of MCI have found that FDG-PET patterns consistent with AD will predict progression to AD, and such predictive power is increased when combined with genetic risk information.[47]

Imaging also offers promise as a surrogate marker for clinical trials. Quantitative MRI and FDG-PET have been used for this purpose. Perhaps the most promising approach is the new form of PET imaging that provides measures of amyloid senile plaques and tau NFTs, the neuropathological hallmarks of AD that accumulate in cortical brain regions in patients with MCI and AD.[43] Combining several imaging modalities with other genetic risk data and neuropsychological profiles will likely improve diagnostic accuracy and resultant treatment outcomes.

Conclusion

Dementia is a major health care problem that will increase as the population ages. FDG-PET scanning provides a reasonably accurate determination of the cause of dementia early in its course. FDG-PET imaging can differentiate AD from the other causes of dementia and can often detect AD when the clinical diagnosis cannot be made without it. This early detection should result in earlier treatment and better responses to AD treatments. Combining PET or other imaging methods with other genetic risk data provides additional information that indicates subtle brain abnormalities even earlier in the course of age-related memory decline. This approach offers promise in clinical trials of agents designed to slow age-related cognitive decline and delay the onset of clinical AD. The use of new methods to provide a signal of amyloid plaques and tangles also offers promise as a strategy for improving early disease detection and monitoring treatments designed to decrease the accumulation of these lesions.

References

1. Bachman DL, Wolf PA, Linn RT, et al: Incidence of dementia and probable Alzheimer's disease in a general population: the Framingham Study. Neurology 43:515–519, 1993.
2. Small GW, Rabins PV, Barry PP, et al: Diagnosis and treatment of Alzheimer's disease and related disorders: consensus statement of the American Association for Geriatric Psychiatry, the Alzheimer's Association, and the American Geriatrics Society. JAMA 78:1363–1371, 1997.
3. Petersen RC, Parisi JE, Dickson DW, et al: Neuropathology of amnestic mild cognitive impairment. Arch Neurol 63:665–672, 2006.
4. Petersen RC, Smith GE, Waring SC, et al: Mild cognitive impairment: clinical characterization and outcome. Arch Neurol 56:303–308, 1999.
5. Andersen K, Nielsen H, Lolk A, et al: Incidence of very mild to severe dementia and Alzheimer's disease in Denmark: the Odense Study. Neurology 52:85–90, 1999.
6. National Institute on Aging: Progress Report on Alzheimer's Disease 1996 (NIH Publ No 96-4137). Bethesda, MD, National Institute on Aging, 1996.
7. Ernst RL, Hay JW: The U.S. economic and social costs of Alzheimer's disease revisited. Am J Public Health 84:1261–1264, 1994.
8. Grundman M, Petersen RC, Ferris SH, et al: Mild cognitive impairment can be distinguished from Alzheimer disease and normal aging for clinical trials. Arch Neurol 61:59–66, 2004.
9. Callahan CM, Hendrie HC, Tierney WM: Documentation and evaluation of cognitive impairment in elderly primary care patients. Ann Intern Med 122:422–429, 1995.
10. Ross GW, Abbott RD, Petrovich H, et al: Frequency and characteristics of silent dementia among elderly Japanese-American men. The Honolulu-Asia Aging Study. JAMA 277:800–805, 1997.
11. Saunders AM, Strittmatter WJ, Schmechel D, et al: Association of apolipoprotein E allele E4 with late-onset familial and sporadic Alzheimer's disease. Neurology 43:1467–1472, 1993.
12. Corder EH, Saunders AM, Strittmatter WJ, et al: Gene dose of apolipoprotein E type 4 allele and the risk of Alzheimer's disease in late onset families. Science 261:921–923, 1993.
13. Relkin NR, Tanzi R, Breitner J, et al: Apolipoprotein E genotyping in Alzheimer's disease: position statement of the National Institute on Aging/Alzheimer's Association Working Group. Lancet 347:1091–1095, 1996.
14. Blennow K, Skoog I: Genetic testing for Alzheimer's disease: how close is reality? Curr Opin Psychiatry 112:487–493, 1999.

15. DeCarli C, Kaye JA, Horwitz B, et al: Critical analysis of the use of computer-assisted transverse axial tomography to study human brain in aging and dementia of the Alzheimer's type. Neurology 40:872–883, 1990.

16. Braak H, Braak E: Neuropathologic staging of Alzheimer-related changes. Acta Neuropathol (Berl) 82:239–259, 1991.

17. Laakso MP, Soininen H, Partanen K, et al: MRI of the hippocampus in Alzheimer's disease: sensitivity, specificity, and analysis of the incorrectly classified subjects. Neurobiol Aging 19:23–31, 1998.

18. Jack CR Jr, Petersen RC, Xu YC, et al: Prediction of AD with MRI-based hippocampal volume in mild cognitive impairment. Neurology 52:1397–1403, 1999.

19. Silverman DHS, Small GW, Phelps ME: Clinical value of neuroimaging in the diagnosis of dementia: sensitivity and specificity of regional cerebral metabolic and other parameters for early identification of Alzheimer's disease. Clin Positron Imaging 2:119–130, 1999.

20. Small GW, Mazziotta JC, Collins MT, et al: Apolipoprotein E type 4 allele and cerebral glucose metabolism in relatives at risk for familial Alzheimer disease. JAMA 273:942–947, 1995.

21. Imamura T, Ishii K, Sasaki M, et al: Regional cerebral glucose metabolism in dementia with Lewy bodies and Alzheimer's disease: a comparative study using positron emission tomography. Neurosci Lett 235:49–52, 1997.

22. Albin RL, Minoshima S, D'Amato CJ, et al: Fluoro-deoxyglucose positron emission tomography in diffuse Lewy body disease. Neurology 47:462–466, 1996.

23. Ishii K, Sakamoto S, Sasaki M, et al: Cerebral glucose metabolism in patients with frontotemporal dementia. J Nucl Med 39:1975–1988, 1998.

24. Mazziotta JC, Phelps ME, Pahl JJ, et al: Reduced cerebral glucose metabolism in asymptomatic subjects at risk for Huntington's disease. N Engl J Med 316:357–362, 1987.

25. Vander Borght T, Minoshima S, Giordani B, et al: Cerebral metabolic differences in Parkinson's and Alzheimer's diseases matched for dementia severity. J Nucl Med 38:797–802, 1997.

26. Silverman DHS, Small GW, Chang CY, et al: Positron emission tomography in evaluation of dementia: regional brain metabolism and long-term clinical outcome. JAMA 286:2120–2127, 2001.

27. Minoshima S, Frey KA, Koeppe RA, et al: A diagnostic approach in Alzheimer's disease using three-dimensional stereotactic surface projections of fluorine-18-FDG PET. J Nucl Med 36:1238–1248, 1995.

28. Chételat G, Desgranges B, de la Sayette V, et al: Mild cognitive impairment: can FDG-PET predict who is to rapidly convert to Alzheimer's disease? Neurology 60:1374–1377, 2003.

29. Kennedy AM, Frackowiak RSJ, Newman SK, et al: Deficits in cerebral glucose metabolism demonstrated by positron emission tomography in individuals at risk of familial Alzheimer's disease. Neurosci Lett 186:17–20, 1995.

30. Reiman EM, Caselli RJ, Yun LS, et al: Preclinical evidence of Alzheimer's disease in persons homozygous for the ε4 allele for apolipoprotein E. N Engl J Med 334:752–758, 1996.

31. Small GW, Ercoli LM, Silverman DHS, et al: Cerebral metabolic and cognitive decline in persons at genetic risk for Alzheimer's disease. Proc Natl Acad Sci U S A 97:6037–6042, 2000.

32. Reiman EM, Caselli RJ, Chen K, et al: Declining brain activity in cognitively normal apolipoprotein E ε4 heterozygotes: a foundation for using positron emission tomography to efficiently test treatments to prevent Alzheimer's disease. Proc Natl Acad Sci USA 98:3334–3339, 2001.

33. Mega MS, Cummings JL, O'Connor SM, et al: Cognitive and metabolic responses to metrifonate therapy in Alzheimer's disease. Neuropsychiatry Neuropsychol Behav Neurol 14:63–68, 2001.

34. Bookheimer SY, Strojwas MH, Cohen MS, et al: Brain activation in older people at genetic risk for Alzheimer's disease. N Engl J Med 343:450–456, 2000.

35. Ashburn TT, Han H, McGuinness BF, et al: Amyloid probes based on Congo Red distinguish between fibrils comprising different peptides. Chem Biol 3:351–358, 1996.

36. Klunk WE, Debnath ML, Pettegrew JW: Chrysamine-G binding to Alzheimer and control brain: autopsy study of a new amyloid probe. Neurobiol Aging 16:541–548, 1995.

37. Lovat LB, O'Brien AA, Armstrong SF, et al: Scintigraphy with ^{123}I-serum amyloid P component in Alzheimer disease. Alzheimer Dis Assoc Disord 12:208–210, 1998.

38. Majocha RE, Reno JM, Friedland RP, et al: Development of a monoclonal antibody specific for beta/A4 amyloid in Alzheimer's disease brain for application to in vivo imaging of amyloid angiopathy. J Nucl Med 33:2184–2189, 1992.

39. Shoghi-Jadid K, Small GW, Agdeppa ED, et al: Localization of neurofibrillary tangles (NFTs) and beta-amyloid plaques (APs) in the brains of living patients with Alzheimer's disease. Am J Geriatr Psychiatry 10:24–35, 2002.

40. Agdeppa ED, Kepe V, Liu J, et al: Binding characteristics of radiofluorinated 6-dialkylamino-2-naphthylethylidene derivatives as positron emission tomography imaging probes for β-amyloid plaques in Alzheimer's disease. J Neurosci 21:RC189, 2001.

41. Klunk WE, Engler H, Nordberg A, et al: Imaging brain amyloid in Alzheimer's disease with Pittsburgh Compound-B. Ann Neurol 55:306–319, 2004.

42. Verhoeff NPLG, Wilson AA, Takeshita S, et al: In-vivo imaging of Alzheimer disease β-amyloid with [^{11}C]SB-13 PET. Am J Geriatr Psychiatry 12:584–595, 2004.

43. Small GW, Kepe V, Ercoli L, et al: FDDNP-PET scanning of cerebral amyloid and tau deposits in MCI. Paper presented at the American Academy of Neurology Annual Meeting, San Diego, CA, April 4, 2006.

44. Kepe V, Cole GM, Liu J, et al: In vivo [F-18]FDDNP microPET imaging of brain β-amyloid in a transgenic rat model of Alzheimer's disease. Alzheimer's & Dementia 1 (suppl 1):S45, 2005.

45. Agdeppa ED, Kepe V, Petric A, et al: In vitro detection of (S)-naproxen and ibuprofen binding to plaques in the Alzheimer's brain using the positron emission tomography molecular imaging probe 2-(1-{6-[(2-[^{18}F]fluoroethyl)(methyl)amino]-2-naphthylethylidene)malononitrile. Neuroscience 117:723–730, 2003.

46. American Psychiatric Association: Diagnostic and Statistical Manual of Mental Disorders, 4th Edition, Text Revision. Washington, DC, American Psychiatric Association, 2000.

47. Mosconi L, Perani D, Sorbi S, et al: MCI conversion to dementia and the APOE genotype: a prediction study with FDG-PET. Neurology 63:2332–2340, 2004.

9

GENETICS AND DEMENTIA NOSOLOGY

Deborah Blacker, M.D., Sc.D.
Simon Lovestone, Ph.D., M.R.C.Psych.

Genetic research depends on an accurate neuropsychiatric nosology and may one day contribute, through a process of triangulation, to improvements in that nosology. To better understand that process, this chapter reviews genetic data on Alzheimer's disease (AD) and other dementias, the impact of nosology on genetic research, and the impact of genetic research findings on nosology. The focus is on AD, for which more genetic data are available; genetic data on other dementias are briefly reviewed as well. In addition, a separate section reviews the relationship of genetic findings and mild cognitive impairment (MCI), a boundary zone between normal aging and dementia, particularly AD.

Supported by the National Institute on Aging (5 P01 AG4853 and 5R37 MH60009, Dr. Blacker) and the Medical Research Council (Dr. Lovestone).

This chapter is reprinted from Blacker D, Lovestone S: "Genetics and Dementia Nosology." *Journal of Geriatric Psychiatry and Neurology* 19:186–191, 2006. Used with permission.

Background: Genetic Findings on Dementia

ALZHEIMER'S DISEASE GENETICS

There is ample evidence that genetic factors are involved in the development of AD. There is a two- to threefold increased risk in the disease among first-degree relatives of AD patients compared with those of controls.[1,2] Also, age at onset tends to be correlated in families.[3] In general, AD shows complex inheritance, but some rare families—typically late-onset—have autosomal dominant inheritance. Twin studies show greater concordance in monozygotic than dizygotic twins, but monozygotic twin concordance is less than 100%, and age at onset may differ by 10 years or more.[4–6] For genetic studies, AD is typically divided into early- and late-onset disease, with age less than 60 years defining early onset. Early-onset cases are more likely to have a positive family history and evidence of autosomal dominant inheritance. Although it was previously thought that only early-onset AD was familial, research in the past two decades has shown that family and twin findings hold in early- and late-onset cases.[6–8]

Four AD genes have been identified. Three cause early-onset AD in an autosomal dominant pattern. The first is the amyloid precursor protein gene *(APP)* on chromosome 21,[9,10] for which 25 mutations affecting 71 families have been reported to date.[11] Age at onset for *APP* mutations is variable and modified by apolipoprotein E *(APOE)* genotype.[12] The second gene is presenilin 1 *(PSEN1)* on chromosome 14,[13,14] for which there are 155 reported mutations affecting 315 families,[11] so most are "genetically private." Onset age for individuals with these mutations is in the 40s and 50s, unaffected by *APOE* genotype,[15] and *PSEN1* accounts for the great majority of autosomal dominant early-onset AD.[16] *PSEN1* mutations are also observed in sporadic early-onset cases.[17] The third gene is presenilin 2 *(PSEN2)* on chromosome 1,[18,19] for which there are 10 reported mutations affecting 18 families.[11] It has a variable age at onset, modified by *APOE* genotype.[20]

The last AD gene is *APOE*,[21,22] a susceptibility gene for AD. *APOE* has three alleles, ε2, ε3, and ε4, with a complex relationship to risk for AD and cardiovascular disease (see Table 9–1).[23–26] The peak impact of the *APOE* ε4 risk allele is in the 60s[23] and decreases markedly after age 80 or 90.[25] *APOE*'s principal effect appears to be as a modifier of age at onset,[27] which falls with the number of copies of the ε4 risk allele.[23,28] Both risk and age-at-onset effects are much greater for *APOE* ε4 homozygotes. Estimates of the magnitude of the *APOE* ε4 effect vary widely (two- to eightfold), probably related to ascertainment issues, because *APOE* effect varies with age (peak in 60s), gender (greater in women), and ethnicity (greater in whites).[23]

Multiple lines of evidence point to the existence of additional AD genes. A segregation analysis predicts four to seven additional AD genes.[29] Family and twin findings hold even after *APOE*[1,4] is controlled for. Despite this, these genes have

TABLE 9–1. Impact of the apolipoprotein E gene (*APOE*) on Alzheimer's disease (AD) risk, cardiovascular risk, and longevity[23–26]

Allele	Frequency	AD risk	Cardiovascular risk	Longevity
2	0.08	Decreased	Decreased	Increased
3	0.78	—	—	—
4	0.16	Increased	Increased	Decreased

been very hard to track down. Although there are multiple association reports (and nonreplications) across the genome, mostly from case–control studies, only *APOE* is definitively associated with AD.[30–32]

GENETICS OF OTHER DEMENTIAS

For other dementias, on the whole there is much less genetic information than for AD. However, for frontotemporal dementia (FTD), extensive new data from genetic and a wide range of other studies have accumulated that suggest a broader syndrome than currently recognized in the *Diagnostic and Statistical Manual of Mental Disorders,* 4th Edition (DSM-IV).[33] FTD is notably familial, and studies suggest that 25%–50% of FTD patients have a first-degree relative with FTD.[34] Many such patients report a family history consistent with autosomal dominant inheritance. Mutations in tau (*MAPT* on chromosome 17),[35] the protein found in the neurofibrillary tangles characteristic of FTD and other neurodegenerative diseases, including AD, are found in 10%–30% of FTD patients with a family history and can be detected in up to 70% of autosomal dominant families.[34,36] Families with *MAPT* mutations often have FTD accompanied by motor syndromes such as Parkinson's disease or predominantly motor disorders with little or no dementia such as progressive supranuclear palsy. A total of 40 such mutations have been reported across 113 families.[11] Just as *MATP* mutations are phenotypically diverse, FTD is genetically heterogeneous,[11] and some families with FTD have mutations also in *PSEN1*[37] and in the chromatin-modifying protein 2B gene *(CHMP2B).*[38]

Creutzfeldt–Jakob dementia (CJD) can also be familial: 15% of cases have a positive family history, typically autosomal dominant. Mutations have been identified in the prion protein gene *(PRNP)* in many of these families.[39,40]

Influence of Nosology on Genetic Research

Research aimed at finding genes for AD and other dementias has reached a difficult juncture. Most of the easy autosomal dominant genes and the large-impact risk factor gene *APOE* have been identified, or, in the phrase that has become standard in the genetics community, the "low-hanging fruit" of dementia genetics has been harvested. A wide variety of strategies have been suggested to move forward, but most investigators agree that optimizing the phenotype definition is critically important.

Improved nosology would help genetic studies in several ways. The first is increasing diagnostic specificity: false positives are generally more damaging to genetic research because unaffected participants and those with other/unclear dementias are usually analyzed as "phenotype unknown." On the other hand, mixed cases are less of a concern in genetic studies, and criteria that are optimized for clinical trials or other applications may sacrifice too much sensitivity to avoid mixed cases. The second is increasing diagnostic sensitivity, which is critical because the number of cases drives the power of genetic analysis. The third is decreasing heterogeneity, which can cause a hidden loss of power. Last, an understanding of nosology could improve genetic research by informing the development of "endophenotypes"—measures closer to the underlying genetic mechanisms, such as age- and education-adjusted memory scores or changes in hippocampal volume. This approach is beyond the scope of discussion of improvements in categorical diagnosis in DSM but may be more productive for finding genes.

ALZHEIMER'S DISEASE GENETICS AND NOSOLOGY

For AD, current diagnostic criteria (DSM-IV criteria or the very similar NINCDS/ADRDA criteria[41]) perform fairly well.[42] Using current definitions, the predictive value positive of a diagnosis of probable AD in an academic center is approximately 90%[43] against an autopsy standard.[44] Nonetheless, improvements in the accuracy of diagnosis would still be of great help in genetic studies.

In terms of diagnostic specificity, there are two major issues. The first is indistinct boundaries with other neurodegenerative disorders, particularly FTD and dementia with Lewy bodies (DLB). Improvements in the diagnostic criteria that are more specific about the typical pattern of deficits in AD and that delineate the presence of early, prominent language symptoms and/or behavioral changes in FTD and the presence of fluctuating course, visual hallucinations, and neuroleptic sensitivity in DLB[42,45] would be helpful. The second major area is overlap with vascular or multi-infarct dementia. Vascular dementia is heterogeneous, as are the strokes that contribute to it, and available consensus definitions vary widely, particularly in the extent that they stress clinical versus radiographic evidence for stroke.[42,46,47] Although the diagnostic criteria for AD already exclude a stepwise course and require instead an insidious onset and gradually progressive course, this is insufficient to rule out all dementia with a significant vascular component. The chances of a clear-cut solution based on categorical diagnosis may be limited given the large number of individuals in whom both forms of pathology probably contribute.

As for increasing diagnostic sensitivity, AD is most often missed because of a mixed picture or insufficient symptoms to diagnose dementia. The most common mixed picture is AD and vascular dementia. As noted earlier, this issue will be difficult, if not impossible, to resolve with changes in diagnostic criteria. The issue of insufficient symptoms is also fundamentally problematic. Whereas criteria for MCI have already been proposed[48] that increase the likelihood of progression to AD, there will always be people who neither are normal nor meet such criteria. In addition, there is an inherent problem in late-life disorders in that people carrying susceptibility variants will always be present among clearly normal participants as well; in contrast to diseases of childhood or midlife, it is not possible to identify individuals who are beyond the age of risk for late-onset AD.

As for decreasing heterogeneity, subtypes might be based on family history, age at onset, specific symptoms (e.g., psychosis), or combinations of these. From the genetic point of view, it makes sense to consider early-onset autosomal dominant cases as a specific subtype—for instance, excluding them from efforts to find susceptibility genes. Support for a specifically psychotic subtype is less compelling. However, there is some support for delineating a syndrome of behavioral and psychological symptoms of dementia, which appears to be heritable, particularly for AD.[49–52] It is plausible, perhaps even likely, that such associations are unrelated to the primary disease but are instead susceptibility factors for the occurrence of these symptoms in the context of any neuropsychiatric insult. If so, then increasing nosological specificity will not necessarily contribute to the search for susceptibility variants. Arguably, a looser disease-based nosology, but improved symptom profiling, would be more likely to lead to progress in AD genetics.

OTHER DEMENTIA GENETICS AND NOSOLOGY

As in AD genetic research, progress in understanding the genetics of other dementias will benefit from clearer definitions. In particular, the considerable progress on FTD in the past decade has not yet been implemented in DSM. Several alternative criteria have been proposed.[33,42,53,54] Incorporating the key features that help to identify FTD into the DSM-V criteria will facilitate genetic and other research. For vascular dementia, as noted earlier, issues with diagnostic criteria are more problematic. Progress in understanding genetics of vascular cognitive impairment and stroke is more likely to come from more careful delineation of stroke subtypes and may require a quantitative approach.

Impact of Genetic Research on Nosology

With a summary of genetic data, and the needs of genetic research laid out, what then can we say about how genetic research can inform an updated nosology of dementia? We review here whether genetic data justify a shift in criteria or definition of formal subtypes for AD and other dementias. We also discuss whether genetic testing or profiling might be used to improve diagnosis and whether there is reason to include genetic tests in the diagnostic criteria.

GENETICS AND THE DIAGNOSIS OF ALZHEIMER'S DISEASE

Genetic data provide no evidence for a shift in the diagnostic criteria for AD. However, as noted earlier, they do validate more careful exclusion of a symptom pattern typical of FTD, a key priority for DSM-V.

There is also limited evidence for AD subtyping based on genetic data. Early-onset cases overall are more likely to have a positive family history and to harbor a mutation in one of the early-onset genes.[16,17] but are clinically indistinguishable from more typical AD. In addition, there is a substantial *APOE* effect in the late 50s through the 60s,[23] which would argue against an arbitrary break at age 60. However, a subtype of autosomal dominant early-onset AD might be useful because these cases have a distinctive picture from the genetic point of view, as well as specific clinical issues growing out of the onset age and family history. It does not make sense to base a diagnosis on specific genes such as *PSEN1*, because some of the mutations in this gene have been associated with non-AD syndromes.[11] There is no support for subtyping of familial versus sporadic cases: family history depends on family size, longevity, and information quality. Support for a subtype based on psychotic symptoms is also limited, at least from the genetic point of view,[49,50–52] although clearly the presence of psychotic symptoms has critical clinical implications.

Despite all the progress in genetic understanding, genetic testing has limited utility in the diagnosis of AD. For early-onset AD, genetic tests add little to diagnosis given the high prior probability of disease in the autosomal dominant setting. However, some clinicians use them to identify the mutation in a particular family, which can then be made available for predictive testing in relatives.[40,55] Overall, genetic testing is complex; however, because of the extensive locus, allelic, and phenotypic heterogeneity (three known genes with nearly 200 different mutations and some variability in phenotype),[11] the yield is higher in families with a high likelihood of *PSEN1* (generally with onset before age 50). *PSEN1* is also the only one of the early-onset genes for which genetic testing is commercially available. Because mutations tend to be "genetically private" (i.e., only one to several families share a given specific mutation), genetic testing generally involves sequencing the gene rather than testing for a specific variant.

For late-onset AD, *APOE* testing can increase the specificity of a clinical diagnosis of AD modestly, but at the expense of decreased sensitivity,[43] and it is not recommended as part of a diagnostic evaluation.[42] There is a broad consensus in the field that *APOE* testing is not appropriate for predictive use because of its poor predictive value.[56–58] However, should a more effective preventive treatment emerge, particularly one with significant cost or side effects, it is conceivable that *APOE* testing might be used as a mechanism to identify individuals at higher risk of subsequent AD for intervention.

GENETICS AND CRITERIA FOR OTHER DEMENTIAS

For FTD, family and genetic data confirm the distinctive symptoms, variable neuropathology, and earlier onset age identified in phenomenological and clinico-pathological studies. To bring DSM in line with current thinking in this area, it is critical to broaden the nomenclature to encompass the wider range of neuropathology now recognized, rather than focus more narrowly on Pick's disease.[33,42] It is also essential to refine the diagnostic criteria to more clearly delineate FTD from AD by focusing on the temporal course of changes in specific domains. As for subtyping, genetic information would support a subtype based on an autosomal dominant family history because of the greater likelihood of a *MATP* mutation and of concomitant motor symptoms and because of the special clinical issues involved. For CJD, genetic data offer little to suggest changes in the criteria but would support an autosomal dominant subtype.

Genetic testing for FTD is not recommended for clinical use.[42] However, there is some experience offering predictive testing for family members in which a *MAPT* mutation has been identified.[59] Genetic testing is also not recommended for CJD.[42]

Genetics and Mild Cognitive Impairment

Genetic data also have little to offer the debate about the validity of a diagnosis of MCI.[48,60,61] This boundary diagnosis between normal aging and dementia is clinically useful for coding patients or research participants with memory complaints who have insufficient impairment for a diagnosis of dementia. In this setting, fairly broad criteria are helpful, because patients tend to be heterogeneous and narrow criteria tend to leave some patients unclassified. This is even truer in nonclinical settings, such as a community survey or family study, because symptoms on average are milder and many participants tend to fall short of stringent definitions of MCI.[60,62]

Another use of MCI criteria is the identification of research participants for studies aimed at stopping dementia at its preclinical phase[63]—and identifying patients with similar attributes who might benefit from any effective intervention. This use favors more specific criteria designed to identify those who are more likely to develop dementia in general or AD in particular. To increase the specificity of an MCI diagnosis for an ultimate diagnosis of AD, a variety of strategies have been considered.[48] In particular, the documentation of a clear-cut amnestic component is more predictive of a subsequent diagnosis of AD. Overall, predictive value for subsequent AD increased by rules that increase likelihood of neurodegeneration in general (gradual progression, more significant reported and observed deficits) and AD in particular (predominance of memory problems, limited vascular symptoms/signs). As would be expected, *APOE* ε4 predicts greater risk of progression within a defined period and makes an ultimate diagnosis of AD more likely,[64,65] but only probabilistically. Thus, there is no role for *APOE* genotyping in the diagnosis of MCI or for defining MCI subtypes. However, as noted earlier, it might be used to select participants or patients at higher risk to test a specific intervention.

Overall, genetic research might benefit from both a narrow definition of MCI, which would be used to identify family members or community participants who have not yet developed dementia but who could be considered affected for purposes of genetic analysis, and a broader definition that could be used to identify family members or community participants who should be considered phenotype unknown. For clinical purposes as well, a broad overall definition, with a subtype indicating those who have a high likelihood of progressing to AD, would be the most helpful.

Genetics and the Nosology of the Future

Despite exceptional progress in the past two to three decades, genetics has only meager offerings for DSM-V. Although we can expect to see discoveries of still more genes for AD and other dementing disorders, and perhaps additional, more clearly delineated (but rare) Mendelian syndromes, these are unlikely to make substantial contributions to nosology. Those who expect a gene test or genetic profile that defines AD or another dementia will be sorely disappointed.

References

1. Payami H, Grimslid H, Oken B, et al: A prospective study of cognitive health in the elderly (Oregon Brain Aging Study): effects of family history and apolipoprotein E genotype. Am J Hum Genet 60:948–956, 1997.

2. Farrer LA, O'Sullivan D, Cupples LA, et al: Assessment of genetic risk for Alzheimer's disease among first-degree relatives. Ann Neurol 25:485–493, 1989.

3. Farrer LA, Myers RH, Cupples LA, et al: Transmission and age-at-onset patterns in familial Alzheimer's disease: evidence for heterogeneity. Neurology 38:395–403, 1990.

4. Bergem AL, Engedal K, Kringlen EL: The role of heredity in late-onset Alzheimer disease and vascular dementia: a twin study. Arch Gen Psychiatry 54:264–270, 1997.

5. Breitner JCS, Welsh KA, Gau BA, et al: Alzheimer's disease in the National Academy of Sciences–National Research Council Registry of Aging Twin Veterans, III: detection of cases, longitudinal results and observations on twin concordance. Arch Neurol 52:763–771, 1995.

6   Raiha I, Kaprio J, Kosenvuo M, et al: Alzheimer's disease in twins. Biomed Pharmacother 51:101–104, 1997.

7. Lautenschlager NT, Cupples LA, Rao VS, et al: Risk of dementia among relatives of Alzheimer's disease patients in the MIRAGE study: what is in store for the oldest old? Neurology 46:641–650, 1996.

8. Silverman JM, Li G, Zaccario ML, et al: Patterns of risk in first-degree relatives of patients with Alzheimer's disease. Arch Gen Psychiatry 51:577–586, 1994.

9. Goate AM, Chartier-Harlin MC, Mullan MC, et al: Segregation of a missense mutation in the amyloid precursor protein gene with familial Alzheimer's disease. Nature 349:704–706, 1991.

10. Tanzi R, Gusella JF, Watkins PC, et al: The amyloid beta protein gene: cDNA cloning, mRNA distribution, and genetic linkage near the Alzheimer locus. Science 235:880–884, 1987.

11. Alzheimer Disease & Frontotemporal Dementia Mutation Database. Available at: http://www.molgen.ua.ac.be/ADMutations/default.cfm?MT=1&ML=3&Page=MutBy-Publication. Accessed March 29, 2006.

12. Sorbi S, Nacmias B, Forleo P, et al: Epistatic effect of APP717 mutation and apolipoprotein E genotype in familial Alzheimer's disease. Ann Neurol 38:124–127, 1993.

13. Schellenberg GD, Bird TD, Wijsman EM, et al: Genetic linkage evidence for a familial Alzheimer's disease locus on chromosome 14. Science 258:668–671, 1992.

14. Sherrington R, Rogaev EI, Liang Y, et al: Cloning of a novel gene bearing missense mutations in early familial Alzheimer disease. Nature 375:754–760, 1995.

15. Van Broeckhoven C, Backhovens H, Cruts M, et al: APOE genotype does not modulate age of onset in families with chromosome 14 encoded Alzheimer's disease. Neurosci Lett 169:179–180, 1994.

16. Tanzi RE, Kovacs DM, Kim T-W: The gene defects responsible for familial Alzheimer's disease. Neurobiol Dis 3:159–168, 1996.

17. Rogaeva EA, Fafel KC, Song YQ, et al: Screening for PS1 mutations in a referral-based series of AD cases: 21 novel mutations. Neurology 57:621–625, 2001.

18. Rogaev EI, Sherrington R, Rogaeva EA, et al: Familial Alzheimer's disease in kindreds with missense mutation in a gene on chromosome 1 related to the Alzheimer's disease type 3 gene. Nature 376:775–778, 1995.

19. Levy-Lehad E, Wasco W, Poorkaj P, et al: Candidate gene for the chromosome 1 familial Alzheimer's disease locus. Science 269:973–977, 1995.

20. Wijsman EM, Daw EW, Yu X, et al: APOE and other loci affect age-at-onset in Alzheimer's disease families with PS2 mutation. Am J Med Genet B Neuropsychiatr Genet 132:14–20, 2005.

21. Strittmatter WJ, Saunders AM, Schmechel D, et al: Apolipoprotein E: high avidity binding to β-amyloid and increased frequency of type 4 allele in late-onset familial Alzheimer disease. Proc Natl Acad Sci USA 90:1977–1981, 1993.

22. Saunders AM, Strittmatter WJ, Schmechel D, et al: Association of apolipoprotein E allele ε4 with late-onset familial and sporadic Alzheimer's disease. Neurology 43:1467–1472, 1993.

23. Farrer LA, Cupples LA, Haines JL, et al: Effects of age, sex, and ethnicity on the association between apolipoprotein E genotype and Alzheimer disease. A meta-analysis. APOE and Alzheimer Disease Meta Analysis Consortium. JAMA 278:1349–1356, 1997.

24. Myers RH, Schaefer EJ, Wilson PWF, et al: Apolipoprotein E4 associated with dementia in a population-based study: the Framingham Study. Neurology 45:673–677, 1996.

25. Breitner JCS, Wyse BW, Anthony JC, et al: APOE-ε4 count predicts age when prevalence of AD increases, then declines: the Cache County Study. Neurology 53:321–331, 1999.

26. Corder EH, Saunders AM, Risch NJ, et al: Protective effect of apolipoprotein E type 2 allele for late onset Alzheimer disease. Nat Genet 7:180–184, 1994.

27. Meyer MR, Tschanz JT, Norton MC, et al: APOE genotype predicts when—not whether—one is predisposed to develop Alzheimer disease. Nat Genet 19:321–322, 1998.

28. Corder EH, Saunders AM, Strittmatter WJ, et al: Gene dose of apolipoprotein E type 4 allele and the risk of Alzheimer's disease in late onset families. Science 261:921–923, 1993.

29. Daw EW, Payami H, Nemens EJ, et al: The number of trait loci in late-onset Alzheimer's disease. Am J Hum Genet 66:196–204, 2000.

30. Kamboh MI: Molecular genetics of late-onset Alzheimer's disease. Ann Hum Genet 68:381–404, 2004.

31. Bertram L, Tanzi L: Alzheimer's disease: one disorder, too many genes? Hum Mol Genet 13:R135–R141, 2004.

32. Bertram L, McQueen M, Mullin K, et al: The AlzGene Database. Alzheimer Research Forum. Available at: http://www.alzgene.org. Accessed March 23, 2006.

33. McKhann GM, Albert MS, Grossman M, et al, and the Work Group on Frontotemporal Dementia and Pick's Disease: Clinical and pathological diagnosis of frontotemporal dementia: report of the Work Group on Frontotemporal Dementia and Pick's Disease. Arch Neurol 58:1803–1809, 2001.

34. Bird T, Knopman D, VanSwieten J, et al: Epidemiology and genetics of frontotemporal dementia/Pick's disease. Ann Neurol 54 (suppl 5):S29–S31, 2003.

35. Foster NL, Wilhelmsen K, Sima AAF, et al: Frontotemporal dementia and parkinsonism linked to chromosome 17: a consensus conference. Ann Neurol 41:706–715, 1997.

36. Poorkaj P, Grossman M, Steinbart E, et al: Frequency of tau mutations in familial and sporadic cases of non-Alzheimer dementia. Arch Neurol 58:383–387, 2001.

37. Dermaut B, Kumar-Singh S, Engelborghs S, et al: A novel presenilin 1 mutation associated with Pick's disease but not beta-amyloid plaques. Ann Neurol 55:617–626, 2004.

38. Skibinski G, Parkinson NJ, Brown JM, et al: Mutations in the endosomal ESCRTIII-complex subunit CHMP2B in frontotemporal dementia. Nat Genet 37:806–808, 2005.

39. Gambetti P, Kong Q, Zou W, et al: Sporadic and familial CJD: classification and characterisation. Br Med Bull 66:213–239, 2003.

40. Williamson J, LaRusse S: Genetics and genetic counseling: recommendations for Alzheimer's disease, frontotemporal dementia, and Creutzfeldt-Jakob disease. Curr Neurol Neurosci Rep 4:351–357, 2004.

41. McKhann G, Drachman D, Folstein M, et al: Clinical diagnosis of Alzheimer's disease: report of the NINCDS-ADRDA Work Group under the auspices of Department of Health and Human Services Task Force on Alzheimer's Disease. Neurology 34:939–944, 1984.

42. Knopman DS, DeKosky ST, Cummings JL, et al: Practice parameter: diagnosis of dementia (an evidence-based review). Report of the Quality Standards Subcommittee of the American Academy of Neurology. Neurology 56:1143–1153, 2001.

43. Mayeux R, Saunders AM, Shea S, et al: Utility of the apolipoprotein E genotype in the diagnosis of Alzheimer's disease. New Engl J Med 338:506–511, 1998.

44. Ronald and Nancy Reagan Research Institute of the Alzheimer's Association and National Institute on Aging Working Group: Consensus report of the Working Group on Molecular and Biochemical Markers of Alzheimer's Disease. Neurobiol Aging 19: 109–116, 1998.

45. McKeith IG, Galasko D, Kosaka K, et al: Consensus guidelines for the clinical and pathologic diagnosis of dementia with Lewy bodies (DLB): report of the consortium on DLB international workshop. Neurology 47:1113–1124, 1996.

46. Chui HC, Victoroff JI, Margolin D, et al: Criteria for the diagnosis of ischemic vascular dementia proposed by the State of California Alzheimer's Disease Diagnostic and Treatment Centers. Neurology 42:473–480, 1992.

47. Roman GC, Tatemichi TK, Erkinjuntti T, et al: Vascular dementia: diagnostic criteria for research studies. Report of the NINDS-AIREN International Workshop. Neurology 43: 250–260, 1993.

48. Petersen RC, Smith GE, Waring SC, et al: Mild cognitive impairment: clinical characterization and outcome. Arch Neurol 56:303–308, 1999.

49. Tunstall N, Owen MJ, Williams J, et al: Familial influence on variation in age of onset and behavioural phenotype in Alzheimer's disease. Br J Psychiatry 176:156–159, 2000.

50. Sweet RA, Nimgaonkar VL, Devlin B, et al: Psychotic symptoms in Alzheimer disease: evidence for a distinct phenotype. Mol Psychiatry 8:383–392, 2003.

51. Sweet RA, Nimgaonkar VL, Devlin B, et al: Increased familial risk of the psychotic phenotype of Alzheimer disease. Neurology 58:907–911, 2002.

52. Bacanu SA, Devlin B, Chowdari KV, et al: Heritability of psychosis in Alzheimer disease. Am J Geriatr Psychiatry 13:624–627, 2005.

53. Neary D, Snowden JS, Gustafson L, et al: Frontotemporal lobar degeneration: a consensus on clinical diagnostic criteria. Neurology 51:1546–1554, 1998.

54. Clinical and neuropathological criteria for frontotemporal dementia. The Lund and Manchester Groups. J Neurol Neurosurg Psychiatry 57:416–418, 1994.

55. Bird TD: Risks and benefits of DNA testing for neurogenetic disorders. Semin Neurol 19:253–259, 1999.

56. American College of Medical Genetics/American Society of Human Genetics (ACMG/ ASHG) Working Group on ApoE and Alzheimer's Disease: Statement on use of apolipoprotein E testing for Alzheimer's disease. JAMA 274:1627–1629, 1995.

57. National Institute on Aging/Alzheimer's Association (NIA/ADA) Working Group: Apolipoprotein E genotyping in Alzheimer's disease position statement. Lancet 347:1091–1095, 1996.

58. McConnell LM, Koenig LM, Greely HT, et al: Genetic testing and Alzheimer disease: has the time come? Nat Med 4:757–759, 1998.

59. Steinbart EJ, Smith CO, Pookaj P, et al: Impact of DNA testing for early-onset familiar Alzheimer disease and frontotemporal dementia. Arch Neurol 58:1828–1831, 2001.

60. Petersen RC, Bennett D: Mild cognitive impairment: is it Alzheimer's disease or not? J Alzheimers Dis 7:241–245, 2005.

61. Petersen RC, Stevens JC, Ganguli M, et al: Practice parameter: early detection of dementia: mild cognitive impairment (an evidence-based review). Report of the Quality Standards Subcommittee of the American Academy of Neurology. Neurology 56:1133–1142, 2001.

62. Albert MS, Blacker D: Mild cognitive impairment and dementia. Annual Review of Clinical Psychology Vol 2, April 2006.

63. Petersen RC, Thomas RG, Grundman M, et al: Vitamin E and donepezil for the treatment of mild cognitive impairment. N Engl J Med 352:2379–2388, 2005.

64. Petersen RC, Smith GE, Ivnik RJ, et al: Apolipoprotein E status as a predictor of the development of Alzheimer's disease in memory-impaired individuals. JAMA 273:1274–1278, 1995.

65. Tierney MC, Szalai JP, Snow WG, et al: A prospective study of the clinical utility of APOE genotype in the prediction of outcome in patients with memory impairment. Neurology 46:149–154, 1996.

INDEX

*Page numbers printed in **boldface** type refer to tables or figures.*